RENAL CELL CARCINOMA

Edited by **Hendrik Van Poppel**

Renal Cell Carcinoma
Edited by Hendrik Van Poppel

Published by InTech
Janeza Trdine 9, 51000 Rijeka, Croatia

Publishing Process Manager Adriana Pecar

Technical Editor Teodora Smiljanic

Cover Designer InTech Design Team

Additional hard copies can be obtained from orders@intechopen.com

Renal Cell Carcinoma, Edited by Hendrik Van Poppel
p. cm.
ISBN 978-953-307-844-1

For EU product safety concerns:
IN TECH d.o.o., Prolaz Marije Krucifikse Kozulić 3, 51000 Rijeka, Croatia,
info@intechopen.com or visit our website at intechopen.com.

Meet the editor

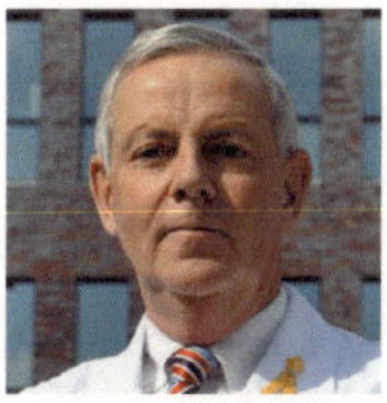

Professor Dr. Hendrik Van Poppel is the Chairman of the Department of Urology at the University Hospital Gasthuisberg, Katholieke Universiteit (KU) Leuven. He graduated in General Surgery in 1980, in Urology in 1983 and joined the Academic Unit at KU Leuven after his postgraduate training in London, Barcelona, Copenhagen, Mainz and Rotterdam. He obtained a PhD in Medical Sciences in 1988, became a Fellow of the European Board of Urology in 1992, and a full Professor of Urology in 1993. Professor Van Poppel is a Board Member of the European Association of Urology (EAU), Chairman of the Educational Office of the EAU and Director of the European School of Urology. He is also a member of the American Association of Genito-Urinary Surgeons, Chairman of the Scientific Committee of Europa Uomo, and Faculty Member of the European Society of Medical Oncology. In addition to that, he is a member of the most prominent urological societies worldwide. Professor Van Poppel has published more than 250 papers as first author and has co-authored more than 270 additional publications on urologic oncology. He is a reviewer for all major urological journals.

Contents

Preface

There is an obvious increase in diagnosis of renal cell carcinoma due to the widespread use of imaging, and it now constitutes 4 % of cancer in adults. Nevertheless, we have been unable to decrease renal cell carcinoma mortality for uncertain reasons, although a lot of progress was made in diagnosis and imaging, recognition of different genetic and pathological entities, management of localized disease (from active surveillance over conventional surgery to minimal invasive techniques), as well as in research on new drug treatments for advanced stages of the disease, potentially combined with surgery. The purpose of this book, which tackles a number of separate interesting topics, is to provide further insight into the disease and the management of early and advanced renal cell carcinoma.

The volume is divided into different parts; the first part covers the characterization of renal masses with imaging, and the second part covers pathology, highlighting a rare distinct entity next to the well-known RCC classification. In the management section, active surveillance, partial nephrectomy and radiofrequency ablation are presented. A separate chapter reports on the state of the art management of Von Hippel Lindau disease, and in the final chapter, conventional and aberrant signaling pathways are explored as possible targets for therapy.

In the first section on imaging and characterization of renal masses, histopathologic and clinical nature of different subtypes of renal masses is outlined. The information on characteristics of these lesions on advanced imaging are synthesized and are of great value in the management decision making. The authors discuss the different renal tumor types, their natural history, their imaging characteristics and demonstrate how imaging can be used in conjunction with other diagnostic tools to optimally characterize renal masses.

The second chapter describes a rare distinct pathological entity of renal cell carcinoma, namely the tubulocystic carcinoma, originally described as a subtype of collecting duct carcinoma but rather low grade. Since tubulocystic carcinoma is not yet included in the current WHO classification it deserves special attention from uropathologists and the treating urologists.

Although we are unable to decrease renal cell carcinoma mortality, there is an ever growing interest in active surveillance of renal cortical neoplasm and its popularity is increasing, probably because more and more small tumors are incidentally detected. Some of them can be benign lesions, but others will definitely be renal cell carcinoma and therefore knowledge of the natural history of these small renal masses is important. The concept of active surveillance of patients with a reduced life expectancy or with a high risk general health status that could make any surgical procedure hazardous is an interesting one. The place of renal biopsy once such a conservative approach is contemplated will be discussed.

Nonetheless, surgical removal of renal masses remains the gold standard, and in the next chapter, the dramatic impact of total nephrectomy on kidney function and on cardiovascular consequences will be highlighted using a hereditary renal cancer population managed at the NCI. The authors show that partial nephrectomy is functionally prudent and can preserve a maximum of renal function while at the same time being oncologically sound and yielding local control rates comparable to radical nephrectomy. Recent advances in laparoscopic and robot assisted minimal invasive surgery will allow earlier convalescence without the incisional complications seen with open surgical procedures.

The next chapter of the book deals with image guided percutaneous ablation of renal tumors. Although no randomized clinical trial has shown equivalence of thermal ablation as compared to surgery, these techniques have recently evolved and their application is likely to increase in the years to come. In the first paper, the general concepts of percutaneous image guided ablation are discussed, followed by a description of different ablation modalities, like radiofrequency ablation and cryoablation, microwave, laser, irreversible electroporation and high intensity focused ultrasound. The place of image guiding with ultrasound, computed tomography and magnetic resonance imaging is presented and different pre-operative and intra-operative details are discussed. The experience with these ablation modalities seems at least promising.

One of them, namely radiofrequency ablation, is discussed in detail in the next chapter, going back to the history of RFA, generators and electrodes, the mechanism of action and the detailed technical application. Importantly, predictive factors for success, clinical outcomes and follow up schedule are presented. Finally, the authors discuss a couple of future prospects that can be applied in combination with percutaneous ablation that constitutes a new field of investigation.

The following chapter provides a nice overview of renal tumors in general, and more specifically renal cell carcinoma in patients with Von Hippel Lindau disease. The historical aspects, genetic disorders and clinical diagnosis are extensively described. Guidelines for screening and surveillance of patients with Von Hippel Lindau disease and renal tumors, not only renal cell carcinomas but also renal cysts and benign tumors, are discussed. Next to excisional nephron sparing surgery, the newer minimal invasive techniques are also put into perspective.

Finally, in the last chapter, targeted therapy for renal cell carcinoma has been described extensively, starting with the molecular biology underlying RCC. A number of registered drugs, and a number of others that are in the pipeline are discussed in an updated overview. The limitations of the currently available targeted agents are acknowledged, which is a reason why the authors extend their discussion onto new possible targets, combination treatments and treatment sequencing that will become more and more relevant in the near future. Researchers and clinicians will have to work together and develop a collaborative strategy to optimize the use of available agents, as well as continue developing clinical trials in order to raise the success rates of medical treatment of patients with RCC.

We are grateful to all authors and researchers who have contributed to the content of this work on renal cell carcinoma. Their great enthusiasm made coordinating the book and collaborating with the InTech staff to produce this book a great pleasure.

Dr. Hendrik Van Poppel
Director of the European School of Urology,
EAU Board Member,
ICUD Treasurer,
Chairman Dept. of Urology, University Hospitals Leuven,
Belgium

1

Radiologic Imaging of Renal Masses

Vincent G. Bird and Victoria Y. Bird
University of Florida, College of Medicine, Department of Urology and Veteran's Administration Medical Center, Gainesville, Florida USA

1. Introduction

Renal cell carcinoma is the third most common urologic malignancy. In the United States in 2010, 58,000 individuals were diagnosed with renal cell carcinoma, of which approximately, 13,000 died. [1] The European Union has experienced a relative increase of 30% for this malignancy over the past two decades. [2] The countries of central and eastern Europe have among the highest recorded incidence of kidney cancers worldwide, with the highest rates observed in the Czech Republic [3] Incidence of this tumor is increasing, the reasons for which are not entirely understood at the current time. Of concern is that despite advances in localized surgical treatment, mortality rates have not decreased.

It is the very nature of this disease that renal masses have long been considered "to be renal cell carcinoma until proven otherwise." The foundation for characterization of renal masses involves imaging. Of critical importance is whether noninvasive imaging can accurately guide diagnosis so as to properly identify those who need intervention, and those, depending on their individual clinical circumstance, who can be safely observed. This goal, which lays at the foundation of research relating to renal masses, has not yet been achieved. Nonetheless, significant advances in understanding of tumor biology have now clarified that renal cell carcinoma is composed of a group of heterogeneous malignancies with distinct genetic abnormalities and natural histories. Advances in imaging technology and techniques has also aided in differentiating benign renal lesions from their malignant counterparts. This new collective understanding of renal masses has given new impetus to more specific characterization of renal masses. This new understanding also allows for a new perspective on the fundamental nature of renal masses that may in turn lead to more precise image based characterization.

1.1 Nature of renal masses

Renal masses are now commonly found as incidental lesions on imaging studies done for other indications. However, review of large series demonstrate that renal masses, notably clinical stage 1 (less than 7.0 cm), are quite heterogeneous. In consideration of this group of renal masses, approximately 20% of them will be benign, with only 20-25% of those that are renal cell carcinoma demonstrating potentially aggressive kidney cancer at time of diagnosis. [4,5,6,7] These renal masses are most commonly diagnosed on abdominal imaging, whether in the form of ultrasound, computerized tomography, or magnetic resonance imaging.

Table 1 summarizes the overall nature of renal masses in the adult population in terms of histological type. Frequency of these lesions is variable, dependant on criteria used for assessing and compiling data. As is the case for many organ systems, though a number of rare uncommon entities are at times found at time of treatment, the focus of the current discussion is on those entities most commonly found. Surgical series may omit patients not candidates for surgery or not desiring intervention. These series may also exclude masses seen on imaging not reaching surgical interventional criteria by the individual investigator. Imaging series may lack complete histopathologic corroboration of all of the lesions noted if not all patients with said lesions underwent treatment where tissue would then be available for histopathologic evaluation. As aforementioned, in many compiled series, notably those focusing on smaller renal masses and associated nephron-sparing procedures, the incidence of benign lesions ranges 20-25%, which is not insignificant.

Renal cyst Simple Complex (Bosniak II, III, and, IV)
Cystic nephroma
Adenoma
Oncocytoma
Angiomyolipoma
Nephroblastoma (Wilm's Tumor)
Transitional cell carcinoma
Renal cell carcinoma Clear cell Papillary Granular Chromophobe Collecting duct Sarcomatoid Renal medullary
Metastases
Other Sarcomas Hemangiopericytoma Leiomyoma

Table 1. Renal Masses

Nonetheless; patients with advanced symptoms still at time times present with higher stage disease. Larger renal masses (greater than 4 cm) are often malignant forms of renal cell carcinoma and are less of a diagnostic dilemma [9]. Moreover, larger renal masses, regardless of nature, have often already compromised a large portion of underlying renal architecture so as to make any meaningful renal salvage unlikely. In contrast, due to their heterogeneous nature, characterization of small masses is of great importance in that such image related information can better stratify patients for different management options. It is likely those with relatively small benign tumors can be spared surgical intervention. Those with tumors of low malignant potential, if having concomitant significant medical co-morbidity and limited life expectancy may potentially be candidates for active surveillance, and those that are generally considered good surgical candidates, can undergo definitive treatment [10]. Though a large number of well accepted possible surgical interventions, many minimally invasive, now exist for treatment of these masses, these procedures are associated with a degree of patient risk, both in terms of surgical-perioperative risks, and longer term risks associated with potential loss of renal function. To date, there remains question as to overall impact on renal function in procedures where partial nephrectomy takes place under renal ischemia.

1.2 Imaging of renal masses

A number of reports in the radiologic literature suggest that Hounsfield attenuation value and enhancement patterns of renal tumors on computerized tomography may be a valuable non-invasive technique to help distinguish both benign tumors and the different subtypes of renal cell carcinoma. [11, 12] This is already often the case for angiomyolipomas, which due to their fat content, are often readily identified and assigned a radiologic diagnosis. Nonetheless, a small percentage of angiomyolipomas are fat poor, and thus elude diagnosis by this means.

To date, techniques and analyses of computerized tomographic data have generally not provided a reliable means of differentiation between oncocytoma and RCC. However, more recent findings suggest that image based characterization, namely by means of differential enhancement characteristics seen on computerized tomography, may indeed aid in the differentiation of benign and malignant renal masses. [13] This is in part due to newer generation scanners for performance of computerized tomography (CT), which can accomplish more data acquisition-related tasks in a relatively shorter period of time. It is also in part due to looking at the image-related characteristics of these lesions in a new or different perspective.

1.3 Renal tumor characteristics

There are a number of tumor characteristics that may aid in their more specific identification by imaging techniques. Such features include size, location, gross morphology, fat content, degree of vascularity (generally relative to the surrounding normal renal parenchyma), nature of vascularity (i.e. rate that contrast is taken up and eliminated from the tumor), growth rate, and a large number of antigenic/cell specific characteristics which may be amenable to specific radiolabelling. A number of studies have been performed with the aim of identifying clinical parameters that may better suggest the benign or malignant nature of a renal mass. These studies suggest that in addition to smaller tumor size- age, female gender, cystic nature, no associated gross hematuria, non-smoking history, and peripheral nature are all more associated with benign masses. [14, 15, 16] Nonetheless, these clinical findings are without a high enough degree of certainty for confirming or ruling out malignant tumor.

This chapter will explore the unique features of different renal masses and the strengths and weakness of different imaging modalities. As is often the case, different imaging modalities offer a unique perspective on characteristics of any given renal mass. The developing role of nuclear medicine for detection of tumor through metabolic characteristics will also be explored. Indeed it may be the case that a constellation of image-related findings may be useful for specific non-invasive characterization of a renal mass, and as such may preclude invasive interventions or further guide management for the patient.

The aims of this discussion are to outline the histopathologic and clinical nature of different subtypes of renal masses, to synthesize this information with characteristics of these lesions seen on advanced abdominal imaging, and to shed light on a means for pre-operative, and possibly non-invasive characterization of these lesions. Such information is of great value to patients with renal masses in terms of assessment of overall risk and decision-making.

2. Features of renal cysts, angiomyolipoma, oncocytoma, and renal cell carcinoma

Though there are a relatively large number of different entities that manifest as renal masses in the adult population, the majority that are common in clinical practice are only of a few types, namely renal cysts, complex renal cysts, angiomyolipoma, oncocytoma, and the histopathologic types of renal cell carcinoma. Moreover, little data exists regarding the more rare entities that manifest as renal masses, and as such, the establishment of general principles regarding their nature is not possible at the current time. As such the attention of this discussion is focused on those more common entities.

2.1 Renal cysts

Though the majority of cysts noted on imaging are simple renal cysts, there is a variety of complex cystic masses, which are to a degree indeterminate in nature, as their probability of harboring malignancy is at times difficult to predict. As such, this matter merits significant attention.

Evidence based classification schemes, based on specific image related findings, have been devised in order to help both physicians and patients understand the relative probability that any given cystic mass may harbor malignant renal tumor. Bosniak first introduced his classification of renal cysts in 1986, and has since made refinements in its use. [17] The Bosniak classification system for renal cysts was first developed based on CT findings. However, it has been applied to other imaging modalities; namely ultrasonography and magnetic resonance imaging (MRI). Bosniak did not recommend that ultrasonography be relied upon for differentiation of surgical from nonsurgical complex cystic renal masses. However, he stated that MRI is useful for characterizing complex cystic renal masses because lesion vascularity, manifesting as enhancement, can be evaluated. The Bosniak classification has been applied to MRI in a reliable manner. [18]

The Bosniak classification system has been widely used by both urologists and radiologists due to its clinical practicality. The currently used classification scheme is shown in table 2. [37] Using the lesion's morphology and enhancement characteristics, each cystic renal lesion can be categorized into one of five groups (categories I, II, IIF, III, and IV) each with associated recommendations for patient treatment. [19, 20, 21, 22] Recent modifications include the use of the IIF category. Follow-up study has shown that many lesions that are well marginated, contain multiple hairline thin septa, have minimal smooth thickening of their wall or septa without measurable enhancement, or contain calcifications, which can be thick, nodular, and irregular, are often benign and as such can be followed. [23] Upon follow-up imaging, any further changes in findings for the lesion in question may then require surgical intervention. Follow-up study has also shown that presence of thick, nodular, and irregular calcification is not as significant as once thought. Rather, it is the presence of associated enhancement that increases risk of malignancy in such lesions. [23, 24]) The critical parameter in the Bosniak classification system is the presence of enhancement, that is to say, presence or absence of tissue vascularity, which generally manifests on imaging as enhancement. The association of this finding with malignant cystic lesions had been the chief reason why many felt that standard ultrasonography alone is not adequate in the evaluation of such lesions. Category III and IV lesions are mainly characterized by enhancement. Nonetheless, with the advent of contrast enhanced renal ultrasound, this issue is now under further investigation.

The goal of the Bosniak classification scheme is to identify those cystic masses with a reasonably high probability of being malignant and thus minimizing the number of benign renal masses that are removed. Category II lesions are generally benign, and can be followed with periodic renal imaging. Statistical probability for malignancy is approximately 50% for category III lesions. Category IV lesions are mostly all malignant tumors. [25]

CATEGORY	DESCRIPTION
I	A benign simple cyst with a hairline thin wall that does not contain septa, calcifications, or solid components. It measures water density and does not enhance.
II	A benign cyst that may contain a few hairline thin septa in which "perceived" enhancement may be present. Fine calcification or a short segment of slightly thickened calcification may be present in the wall or septa. Uniformly high attenuation lesions <3 cm (so-called high-density cysts) that are well marginated and do not enhance are included in this group. Cysts in this category do not require further evaluation.
IIF (F for follow-up)	Cysts that may contain multiple hairline thin septa or minimal smooth thickening of their wall or septa. Perceived enhancement of their septa or wall may be present. Their wall or septa may contain calcification that may be thick and nodular, but no measurable contrast enhancement is present. These lesions are generally well marginated. Totally intrarenal nonenhancing high-attenuation renal lesions >3 cm are also included in this category. These lesions require follow-up studies to prove benignity.
III	"Indeterminate" cystic masses that have thickened irregular or smooth walls or septa in which measurable enhancement is present. These are surgical lesions, although some will prove to be benign (eg, hemorrhagic cysts, chronic infected cysts, and multiloculated cystic nephroma), some will be malignant, such as cystic renal cell carcinoma and multiloculated cystic renal cell carcinoma.
IV	These are clearly malignant cystic masses that can have all the criteria of category III, but also contain enhancing soft-tissue components adjacent to, but independent of, the wall or septum. These lesions include cystic carcinomas and require surgical removal.

Table 2. Bosniak classification for cystic renal masses [19]

Biopsy of a renal mass is often entertained as another means to differentiate surgical from nonsurgical cystic lesions, however there are a number of studies that point to the lack of reliability or need for doing so in the majority of cases pertaining specifically to cystic renal masses.[26, 27, 28, 29, 30] Furthermore, although reportedly rare, biopsy of a neoplastic lesion can cause needle tumor seeding and, in cystic masses, potential spillage and implantation of malignant cells.[14,17] In contrast, biopsy of solid renal masses is quite common, and more so since active surveillance may be a possible management option.

2.2 Renal angiomyolipoma

Angiomyolipomas (AML) are benign neoplasms that, as their name implies, consist of varying amounts of mature adipose tissue, smooth muscle, and blood vessels. [31, 32] It is postulated that angiomyolipomas are derived from the perivascular epithelioid cells.[33] Growth of this neoplasm may be hormone dependent, which is suggested by both its predominance in the female and adult population. [33, 34] 20% to 30% of AMLs are found in patients with tuberous sclerosis syndrome, an autosomal dominant disorder characterized by mental retardation, epilepsy, and adenoma sebaceum (distinctive skin lesion). Of those with tuberous sclerosis, 50% develop renal AML. [33, 34, 35] Renal AML is also more often bilateral and multifocal in this group. In tuberous sclerosis patients renal AML occurs at a 2:1 female: male ratio. [34, 35] In the absence of the tuberous sclerosis complex the lesion occurs more often in female patients, with most patients presenting later in life, during the fifth or sixth decade.[33, 34]

Though non-malignant, renal AML may still be of concern in that they can be associated with serious or fatal hemorrhage. Risk of hemorrhage has been associated with both pregnancy and tumor size. [33, 36]. More than 50% of renal AML are now found incidentally due to more prevalent use of abdominal imaging for the evaluation of a wide variety of nonspecific complaints. [37] On rare occasions these neoplasms may display unusual behavior. Benign AML involving the renal vein and vena cava as a tumor thrombus has been reported. [183]. Further, despite their benign nature, extrarenal occurrences have been reported in renal hilar lymph nodes, retroperitoneum, and liver. Direct extension into the venous system has been reported. A uniformly benign clinical course in such cases has argued in favor of multifocal origin rather than metastasis [33, 38, 32 39]. However, very rare malignant variants of AML have been described.[40, 41] Recent review of this matter suggests that benign AML and more aggressive variants may all arise from perivascular epitheloid cells and that they exist as a spectrum of disease, with the majority having a benign nature. [184, 185]. AML behaving in an irregular manner generally require intense histopathologic scrutiny to ensure proper diagnosis.

2.3 Renal oncocytoma

Literature review suggests that this benign behaving renal histopathologic type represents approximately 3% to 11% of all solid renal masses [42, 43, 44, 45] Mean age at presentation and male-to-female predominance are similar for oncocytoma and RCC, and although oncocytomas are more likely to be asymptomatic (58% to 83%), most RCCs are now also diagnosed incidentally. [46, 44, 42, 47] Mean tumor size for oncocytomas has ranged from 4 to 6 cm in most series-again, similar to RCC. However, giant oncocytomas (16-18 cm) have been reported. [186, 187]. It is important to mindful that even very large lesions may be benign, and that if possible, organ sparing surgery should be a consideration. [48, 49, 50, 51]. Familial renal oncocytomatosis is relatively uncommon, but also has been noted.

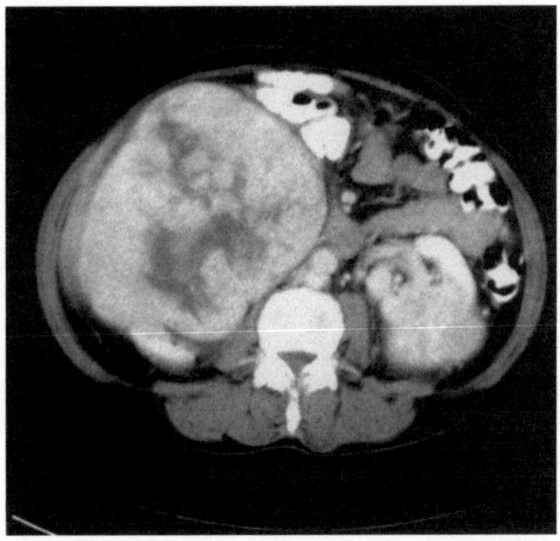

Fig. 1. CT shows 16 x 12 x 15 cm tumor at the caudal pole of the right kidney and 11 x 8.5 12 cm tumor at cranial pole of left kidney. Ponholzer A, Reiter WJ, and Maier U. (2002) Organ sparing surgery for giant bilateral renal oncocytoma. *J. Urol;* 2002: 2531-2532.

In gross appearance, renal oncocytomas are light brown or tan, homogeneous, and well circumscribed tumors. Similar to most renal tumors, they are not truly encapsulated. A central scar may be seen in approximately one third of cases [54], but prominent necrosis is generally not seen. [52, 53] Historically, hypervascularity has been thought to be lacking [52, 53], but these lesions often enhance intensely on contrast enhanced imaging. Oncocytomas cells are packed with numerous large mitochondria, which contributes to their distinctive staining characteristics. Hemorrhage is found in 20% to 30% of cases [44, 54]. Extension into the perinephric fat has also been reported in 11% to 20% of cases, [46, 54] however this is most often not the case in the smaller such lesions that have been resected in recent series. A transitional histopathologic type has been described in the Birt-Hogg-Dubé syndrome, in which renal oncocytomas, chromophobe renal cell carcinoma, and distinctive cutaneous lesions often develop [55]. These transitional neoplasms exhibit features of both oncocytoma and chromophobe RCC, and some authors have hypothesized that there may be a spectrum of tumors spanning both of these histopathologic types [55, 56, 57].

It has long since been known that renal oncocytomas often manifest atypia. However, it has been realized that "atypical"features are part of the renal oncocytoma morphological spectrum and do not appear to affect tumor behavior adversely. [54] Indeed the dilemma of oncocytoma relates to these atypia and its apparent relationship with chromophobe renal cell carcinoma. To date, considerable debate still exists in cases where both of these entities are present. Morphology is often used as the standard. There are a number of reports documenting the coexistence of renal cell carcinomas, not limited to chromophobe RCC, in primary oncocytomas. Though two studies from two referral centers reported a co-existence of 10%-32% [58, 59], a larger number of studies report this incidence to be 0 to 7.2% [54, 60, 61, 62, 63, 64]. This same issue limits the utility of fine-needle aspiration or biopsy [43, 50, 51]. It is possible that evolving molecular and immunohistochemical techniques may further aid in clarification of this issue. Historically, most renal oncocytomas cannot be differentiated from malignant RCC by clinical or radiographic means [65].

2.4 Renal cell carcinoma

Renal cell carcinoma is the most lethal of all urologic cancers, with more than 40% of patients with this malignancy dying of their cancer. It accounts for 2% to 3% of all adult malignant neoplasms. [66, 67, 190] There is a male-to-female predominance of 3:2 [66]. Renal cell carcinoma is primarily a disease of elderly patients, presenting in the sixth and seventh decades of life [67]. The majority of cases of RCC are believed to be sporadic; the United States National Cancer Institute estimates that only 4% are familial. A number of familial conditions associated with renal cell carcinoma are described in the literature. Incidence rates are 10% to 20% higher in African Americans for unknown reasons [68, 190].

The incidence of RCC has increased since the 1970s by an average of 3% per year. This appears in part to be due to the more prevalent use of abdominal imaging for the evaluation of a variety of abdominal, gastrointestinal, and other nonspecific complaints [68]. This trend has correlated with an increased proportion of incidentally discovered and localized tumors and with improved 5-year survival rates for patients with this stage of disease [67, 69]. However, other factors must also be at play because Chow and colleagues [68] have documented a steadily increasing mortality rate from RCC per unit population since the 1980s, and this was observed in all ethnic and both sex groups[191].

Most sporadic RCCs are unilateral and unifocal. However satellite lesions are known to occur, and are often small and difficult to identify by preoperative imaging, intraoperative ultrasonography, or visual inspection; they appear to be the main factor contributing to local recurrence after partial nephrectomy. [70, 71] Bilateral involvement can be synchronous or asynchronous and is found in 2% to 4% of sporadic RCCs, although it is considerably more common in patients with von Hippel-Lindau disease or other familial forms of RCC.[56, 72, 73]. Multifocal disease, which is found in 10% to 20% of cases, is more common in association with papillary histology and familial RCC. [74, 75]

All RCCs were traditionally thought to arise primarily from the proximal convoluted tubules, and this is probably true for most clear cell and papillary variants. However, more recent data suggest that the other histologic subtypes of RCC, such as chromophobe and collecting duct RCC, are derived from the more distal components of the nephron. [76, 77, 78] As of recent, urologic researchers have recognized the distinct nature of the various histopathologic subtypes of RCC through advances in molecular genetics, which has greatly aided in their proper classification.[72]

All RCCs are, by definition, adenocarcinomas, derived from renal tubular epithelial cells [78, 53, 79]. Most RCCs share ultrastructural features, such as surface microvilli and complex intracellular junctions, with normal proximal tubular cells, and they are believed to be derived from this region of the nephron [73]. All of these recent developments indicate that RCC is not a single malignant neoplasm but rather comprises several different tumor subtypes, each with a distinct genetic basis and unique clinical features.

Most RCCs are round to ovoid and circumscribed by a pseudocapsule of compressed parenchyma and fibrous tissue rather than a true histologic capsule. RCCs commonly consist of yellow, tan, or brown tumor interspersed with fibrotic, necrotic, or hemorrhagic areas; they are generally not uniform in gross appearance. Cystic degeneration is found in 10% to 25% of RCCs and appears to be associated with a better prognosis compared with purely solid RCC [88, 89, 90, 91, 190]. Calcification can be stippled or in plaque form, and is found in 10% to 20% of RCCs. Aggressive local behavior is not uncommon with RCC and manifests in a number of ways. Invasion and penetration into the collecting system or renal capsule are found in approximately 20% of cases, although displacement of these structures is more commonly seen. Further local spread to involve adjacent organs or the abdominal wall is often precluded by Gerota's fascia, although some high-grade RCCs may penetrate this barrier. A notable feature of RCC is its occasional involvement of the venous system, which is found in 10% of RCCs, more often than in any other tumor type. [92, 93]

RCC TYPE	PREVALENCE	ORIGIN	KEY FEATURES
Clear cell	70-80%	Proximal tubule	Hypervascular, aggressive behavior common, most likely to have sarcomatoid features
Papillary	10-15%	Proximal tubule	Hypovascular, multifocality is common
Chromophobe	3-5%	Cortical portion of the collecting duct	Prognosis better than conventional Some aggressive variants
Rare	< 1%		
Collecting duct		Collecting duct	Infiltrative, generally aggressive
Medullary		Calyceal epithelium	Infiltrative, generally aggressive, patients with sickle cell trait
Unclassified			Generally aggressive

Table 3. Subtypes of renal cell carcinoma [55, 72, 73, 76, 80, 79]

RCC has long been recognized as one of the most vascular of cancers as reflected by the distinctive neovascular pattern exhibited on renal angiography. Unlike upper tract transitional cell carcinomas, most RCCs are not grossly infiltrative, with the exception of collecting duct RCC and some sarcomatoid variants. [73] Tumors smaller than 3 cm were previously classified as benign adenomas, but some small tumors have been associated with metastases, and most pathologists agree that with the exception of oncocytoma, there are no reliable histologic or ultrastructural criteria to differentiate benign from malignant renal cell epithelial tumors [73].

The vascular nature of RCC plays a special role in imaging of this tumor. Various studies have tried to differentiate between the clear cell and papillary subtypes of RCC based on the degree of enhancement on contrast-enhanced CT as well as MRI. As a general point, a number of these studies have shown excellent accuracy, with higher early enhancement in clear cell renal cancers. [94] In addition, clear cell RCC has a strong association with necrosis and retroperitoneal collateral circulation that is best seen on MRI [95]. On the other hand, papillary RCCs show homogeneous low-level enhancement on both CT and MRI [94, 96]. This will be discussed in detail for each type of imaging modality.

The indications for percutaneous renal biopsy or aspiration in the evaluation of solid renal masses have traditionally been limited, primarily related to concerns about sampling error, difficulty interpreting limited tissue given the inherent similarities between the eosinophilic variants of RCC and oncocytoma, and recognition of the improved diagnostic accuracy of cross-sectional imaging such as CT or MRI. [82, 83] Eighty-three percent to 90% of solid renal masses thought to be suspicious for RCC based on careful radiographic evaluation prove to be RCC on final pathologic analysis [84]. Fine-needle aspiration biopsy (FNAB) cannot significantly improve on this degree of diagnostic certainty and is unlikely to influence clinical management in the majority of cases [27, 85]. More recently, FNAB has been reassessed, and several groups have shown enthusiasm for this approach. Some studies suggest improved sensitivity and specificity, particularly when FNAB is combined with molecular analysis for CA-9 expression or other markers for RCC. Molecular analysis could also assess HMB-45 expression to evaluate for atypical AML, and genetic analysis for oncocytoma may also be available in the near future. In addition, FNAB could influence clinical management of small renal masses if markers of clinical aggressiveness could be established and reliably evaluated on limited pathologic material. The potential complications of FNAB include bleeding, infection, arteriovenous fistula, needle track seeding, and pneumothorax. [82] In general, the incidence of complications has been reduced significantly since the introduction of smaller gauge needles. Tumor location, operator expertise, and number of biopsy attempts can also influence complication rates. Perinephric bleeding can be detected by CT scan in 90% of cases, but clinically significant hemorrhage resulting in gross hematuria is much less common (5% to 7%) and is almost always self-limited [86, 87]. Only five cases of needle track seeding have been reported with RCC. Overall, the estimated incidence of needle track seeding with urologic malignant neoplasms is less than 0.01%; most occur with poorly differentiated transitional cell carcinoma [82].

3. Imaging modalities

Anatomic imaging modalities historically used for the characterization of renal masses include intravenous contrast-enhanced plain film radiography, ultrasonography, computerized tomography, and magnetic resonance imaging. Imaging via nuclear medicine and hybrid nuclear medicine/computerized tomography techniques has also emerged.

Plain film radiography and computerized tomography require use of ionizing radiation. Advances in radiation technology and equipment design have resulted in lower does and overall exposure, but total exposure is additive. Total exposure to ionizing radiation for a patient is of consideration, as there are carcinogenic risks associated with exposure to large cumulative doses of radiation. Total radiation exposure is measured in a number of different manners. Doses may be measured as both skin doses and total effective radiation dose. Effective absorbed radiation, in Sieverts, can also be measured. Cumulative evidence from a number of studies suggests that three-phase CT scan exposes patients to approximately two to three times as much radiation as approximately 12 plain film radiographs (though not that many be required) taken during the course of intravenous pyelography (IVP). [97, 98, 99] More advanced CT protocols, namely multiphase protocols, have made this issue of more significant concern. Possibilities for limiting radiation in these studies include eliminating a phase (which may then limit examination accuracy) or reducing mA during some of the phases of the study. [100] At the current time, low dose CT protocols are being investigated, primarily in the setting of urinary lithiasis, with a focus on maintaining diagnostic accuracy while decreasing exposure. Patients of higher body mass index may not be ideal for low dose CT [101]. Newer subtraction techniques may also allow for fewer runs through the scanner

Intravenous contrast-enhanced plain film radiography and computerized tomography both also involve the use of intravenous iodinated contrast agents, which carry an albeit low, but real risk. Iodinated contrast media entail risk in three manners: (1) metabolic effect relating to their hypertonicity, (2) inducement of acute renal dysfunction, and (3) idiosyncratic contrast material reactions.

Risks associated with hypertonicity include increased cardiac output and decreased peripheral vascular resistance due to volume expansion [102], inhibition of the coagulation cascade by high osmolar contrast agents [103], and renovascular dilation followed by renovascular constriction, with a result decrease in glomerular filtration rate. [104]
Acute impairment in renal function (increase in serum creatinine of 0.5 to 1.0 mg/dl or 25-50% decrease in GFR) occurs in 1/1,000-5,000 patients without known risk factors. This condition is generally nonoliguric, however, when it is accompanied by oliguria, risk of permanent renal damage exists. [105, 106] Risk factors increasing the risk of acute renal dysfunction include dehydration, pre-existing renal insufficiency, diabetic nephropathy, congestive heart failure, hyperuricemia, proteinuria, and multiple administrations of contrast material in a short time period. [107]. General recommendations to avoid acute renal dysfunction include ample pre-examination hydration, avoidance of dehydrating preparations, and a reduction in total contrast used, if feasible.
Patients taking metformin for control of diabetes mellitus are advised to stop this medication 48 hours prior to contrast administration. When renal function and urine output are demonstrated to be normal after imaging, metformin therapy may be resumed. The concern for these patients is that if acute renal dysfunction occurs during metformin administration, these patients may develop significant lactic acidosis. [108]
Idiosyncratic contrast material reactions may occur in mild, moderate, and severe forms. Mild reactions include metallic taste, sensation of warmth, sneezing, coughing, and mild urticaria. Moderate reactions include vomiting, more severe urticaria, headache, edema, and palpitations. These reactions can be symptomatically treated as needed. However, severe reactions, which include hypotension, bronchospasm, laryngeal edema, pulmonary edema, and loss of consciousness, require immediate intervention. Severe reactions occur in less than 0.1% of patients, and it is estimated that 80% of these may be avoided by use of low osmolar contrast media. [109, 110]
All contrast-associated risks appear to be lowered by use of low osmolar contrast media currently available. Administration of prophylactic corticosteroids and use of low osmolar contrast media have been shown to decrease the risk of contrast reaction, but not eliminate it. [111] Methylprednisolone 32 mg oral may be given every 12 hours starting 24 hours prior to examination. This is continued 12-24 hours after the examination to ensure that all contrast material has been excreted. [112] Diphenhydramine 50 mg oral may also be administered before contrast administration. All patients offered intravenous iodinated contrast studies should be counseled and informed of these associated risks.
Many imaging studies relate to differentiation of benign and malignant lesions. Nonetheless they will be presented in the following where to they relate best to the discussion.

3.1 Contrast-enhanced plain film radiography

The IVP, or intravenous pyelogram (also IVU-intravenous urogram) had long been a mainstay of urologic diagnostic imaging. This test requires use of intravenous iodinated contrast. IVP generally requires bowel preparation for optimal imaging results, an absence of patient contraindications to intravenous iodinated contrast administration, repeated imaging over thirty to sixty minutes, and at times more prolonged imaging if renal obstruction is present.
After a scout film is taken, contrast is injected, at which time nephrotomograms are obtained. These images may reveal abnormalities of the renal parenchyma. However recent

studies comparing IVP to other imaging modalities, namely computerized tomography, show that sensitivity for detection and characterization of renal masses is limited. [113] Findings suggestive of a mass seen on IVP generally require other types of imaging for both corroboration and specific delineation.

IVP may provide valuable information pertaining to the pyelocalyceal system, including the existence of hydronephrosis, hydroureteronephrosis, existence of urinary stones, and "filling defects" which include a variety of diagnostic possibilities. However, IVP has limited sensitivity for renal parenchymal pathologies. Previous studies have documented the limited sensitivity of small renal masses, particularly when masses are less than 3 cm [113, 114, 115, 116]. CT urography has gained great popularity in that it provides reliable assessment of both the renal parenchyma and collecting system. A prospective comparison of contrast enhanced CT and IVP in initial evaluation of microscopic hematuria demonstrated that examination with CT had better diagnostic yield for a wide variety of pathologies. [113]

IVP has fallen out of favor at many institutions for a variety of reasons that include; risk of contrast toxicity, time consumption involved in performance of test, and limited diagnostic accuracy in triage setting where diagnoses are often still uncertain. In many institutions it is now only rarely performed.

3.2 Ultrasonography

Ultrasound requires neither iodinated or gadolinium-based contrast administration, nor ionizing radiation. Its mechanism of action is based on the transmission of a pulse of high frequency sound energy into the patient. These sound waves are then reflected, refracted, or absorbed, depending on type of tissue encountered. The ultrasound transducer also acts as a receiver, which receives the returning echoes. Collected input is processed by a computer for the creation of a composite image. [117] Ultrasound is performed in a real time manner which allows for the technician and physician to modify and review different aspects of the examination. Newer machines also have significantly improved resolution.

Ultrasonography is used widely throughout medicine. It may be used by anyone with proper training and experience in almost any clinical scenario; radiology suite, emergency room, clinic, and under sterile conditions in the operating room. The applications of ultrasonography are so extensive that they are beyond enumeration here. However, it is of critical importance to understand that imaging performed with this modality is operator-dependent. This generally requires that the interpreter of the study be present during the actual real-time study. Image quality is also closely related to the quality of equipment being used.

Ultrasonography is performed with use of a variety of probes depending on parameters that include patient body habitus and structures to be imaged. In the case of the kidney, 3.5 to 5 MHz transducers are typically used. Transducers of this range are used to obtain adequate depth of penetration without substantial loss of resolution. Bony structures and bowel gas may both interfere with renal imaging, more so on the left than the right.

Ultrasound is commonly employed as an initial imaging exam due to its relative low cost, relative ease of performance, and lack of need for ionizing radiation. The strength of ultrasonography is its ability to differentiate solid versus cystic renal structures. In the hands of an experienced ultrasonographer, it is quite reliable for the identification and confirmation of simple renal cysts. Historically, there has been concern regarding low sensitivity for detection of small renal masses. [114. 116] However there is evidence that well

performed duplex ultrasonography may be highly accurate in the diagnosis and staging of a large number of renal masses, including those cases where renal vein or caval thrombus are involved. As active surveillance has become an option for select patients with renal masses, type of surveillance imaging has become an important issue. A recent study comparing size of renal masses noted on US, CT, and MRI, comparing imaging results to final pathology, demonstrated all three modalities accurately predicted pathologic tumor size. This study included relatively small renal masses as well. [118] However, there may be limitations with use of ultrasound in respect to the identification of lymphadenopathy. [119]
Renal ultrasonography also has a large role in imaging in patients with azotemia, those with severe contrast allergy, pregnant patients, neonates, and children. Ultrasonography may at times be quite useful for assessment of renal masses in the intraoperative setting, both for open cases and laparoscopic cases. In the open setting it may be useful for the identification of relatively small masses completely hidden within the renal parenchyma, or in cases where multiple small tumors, not all of which are immediately amenable to manual palpation, are suspected. Laparoscopic ultrasound may be useful in a similar fashion, and may also be used in concert with different ablative devices that are at times used in the treatment of select renal masses. [120]

3.2.1 Advances in ultrasound technology and technique

Concerns with use of renal ultrasound for detection of renal masses is noted from earlier data showing that renal masses 3 cm and less are detected only 67-79% of the time. [121]. One must consider that renal tumors may at times have similar echogenicity to normal renal parenchyma. However, with improvements in ultrasound technology, namely in terms of resolution and Doppler technology, this may no longer be the case. More recently, contrast-enhanced ultrasonography (CEUS) has been introduced as another means of further characterizing renal masses. Ultrasound contrast agents (gas filled microbubbles covered by a stabilizing shell) are injected as liquids, and then manifest as a gas when in the bloodstream. This contrast agent, in its gas form, improves the detection of Doppler signals and helps better reveal both normal and abnormal vascularity. [122] At time of performance of the study, the contrast agent is injected, and when evident on imaging, the patient holds their breath while a number of ultrasound frames are obtained for analysis. CEUS entails less risk than contrast-enhanced computerized tomography, can show even subtle tumor blood flow, and may serve as a viable alternative for patients unable to undergo contrast enhanced CT or MRI for any variety of reasons. [123] In study of complex cystic renal masses CEUS has shown to be comparable in characterization of such masses with use of the Bosniak system. [124, 125] CEUS may also improve visualization of renal vessels, detection of vascularity in solid renal masses, and detection of vascularity in septa and walls of complex renal masses. [126, 127, 128] Use of microbubbles in this manner has been shown to have a high safety profile, with incidence of adverse reactions lower than that observed for iodinated and gadolinium based contrast agents.[129]

3.2.2 Ultrasonography and differentiation of renal masses

Angiomyolipomas most often are associated with distinct radiographic findings, which generally relate to their fat content. The typical but not diagnostic finding of AML on ultrasonography is a well-circumscribed, highly echogenic lesion, often associated with shadowing. [37, 25] The finding of shadowing should suggest an AML rather than a small, echogenic RCC, which rarely shadows [25]. In terms of differentiation and characterization of solid renal masses using ultrasonography, the presence of shadowing, a hypoechoic rim, and intratumoral cysts are thought to be important findings that may help distinguish angiomyolipomas from other solid lesions, namely renal cell carcinoma. [130] Nonetheless, these findings are not reliable enough to make such a diagnosis with reasonable certainty. Although conventional ultrasound has not resulted in more specific characterization of renal masses in terms of histopathologic type/subtype, this will issue will likely be re-evaluated with introduction of CEUS.

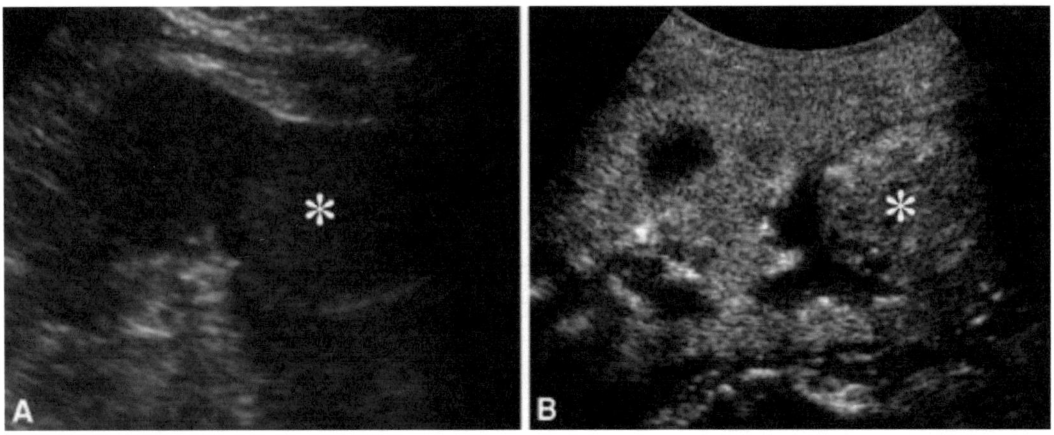

Fig. 2. Renal tumor at the lower pole of the right kidney. Transverse scans. a. A well-defined expansive, hyperechoic mass is observed at grey-scale ultrasound. b. The mass shows intense enhancement at CEUS. Siracusano S, Bertolotto M, Ciciliato S, et al (2011) World J Urol. Epub ahead of print.

3.3 Computerized tomography

Sir Godfrey Newbold Hounsfield, (28 August 1919 - 12 August 2004) and Allan MacLeod Cormack (February 23, 1924 - May 7, 1998) shared the 1979 Nobel Prize for Physiology/ Medicine for developing the diagnostic technique of X-ray computed tomography (CT). Beyond doubt, the introduction of the CT scanner is a critical point in the evolution of medicine.

Since time of inception, CT has taken an increasing role in the realm of imaging. In 2006, over 60 million CT examinations were performed in the United States. [131] In 2008, over 140 million CT examinations were performed worldwide. [132] Similar to plain film radiography, images obtained by this modality are created due to the attenuation of photons by the body tissue being examined. A thin collimated x-ray beam is generated on one side of the patient. Detectors on the opposite side of the patient then measure the amount of transmitted radiation. In any given transverse plane being examined these measurements are repeated as the x-ray beam rotates around the patient. During processing, the measurements are taken and placed into a matrix of CT values that correspond to attenuation of a given tissue volume within the patient. The gray scale of each CT pixel is related to the amount of radiation absorbed at that point. This value is called the attenuation value, and is commonly denoted in Hounsfield units. Clinically relevant CT Hounsfield unit values are shown in table 3. [133, 117]

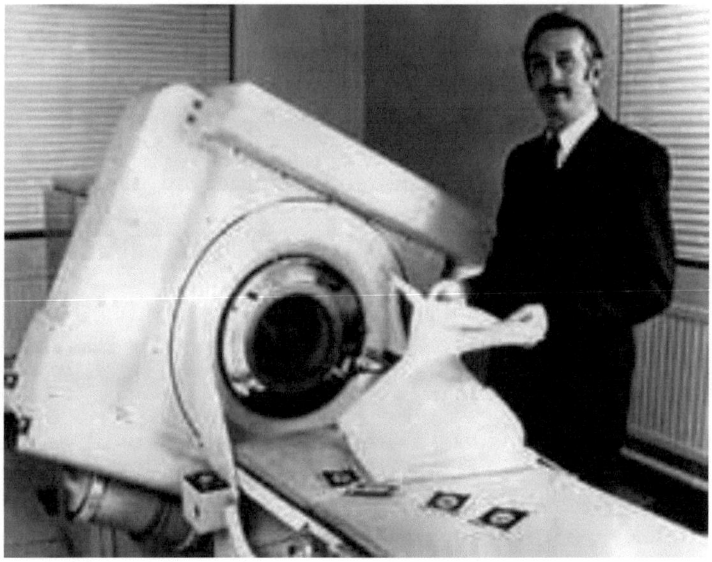

Fig. 3. Sir Godfrey Newbold Hounsfield, (28 August 1919 – 12 August 2004) standing beside early CT scanner. Source: unknown

Absorber	CT numbers (HUs)
Bone	+1000
Calculus	+400 or greater
Calcification	+160 OR GREATER
Acute hemorrhage	+50 to 90
Soft Tissue	+10 to 50
Water	0
Fat	-100
Air	-1000

Table 4. Hounsfield Values [133]

Obtained measurements are then taken from a given transverse slice of body tissue and are mathematically processed by a computer that then reconstructs a cross-sectional image of the body. Early CT scanners obtained transverse images one slice at a time. However, later generation spiral (or helical) CT scanners allow patient movement on a gantry with simultaneous tunnel rotation with continuous x-ray exposure. This arrangement allows for rapid acquisition of volumetric data from the patient being examined during the time in which breathing is suspended. The acquisition of volumetric data is of great value in terms of renal imaging in that it allows for greater accuracy and detail in terms of evaluating renal parenchymal masses and renal vasculature, particularly in terms of visualization of small renal masses and supernumerary renal blood vessels. Studies have indeed shown that thin slice overlapping reconstructions are quite useful for differentiation and accurate depiction for renal masses as small as 5 mm. [188]) Data acquired in this manner also allows for high quality CT angiography and three dimensional reconstructions in a variety of manners. [117]

Contrast enhanced computerized tomography provides excellent anatomic detail for retroperitoneal structures and has become the primary imaging modality for renal masses. Distinct phases have been clearly identified for patients undergoing intravenous contrast-enhanced renal imaging. These phases include the arterial, corticomedullary, nephrographic, and excretory. The arterial phase occurs approximately 15-25 seconds after contrast administration. It is most useful for identification of renal arterial anatomy, evaluating potential renal donors, and those with suspected renovascular pathologies. The corticomedullary phase occurs approximately 25-70 seconds after injection. During this phase the renal cortex has intense enhancement, as glomerular filtration of the contrast material begins to take place. This phase is useful for the identification of hypervascular renal tumors, notably clear cell renal cell carcinomas. The renal veins can also be seen well during this phase. The nephrographic phase generally occurs 80-120 seconds after contrast administration. During this phase contrast has been filtered through the glomeruli and has made its way to the collecting ducts. During this phase the renal parenchyma appears homogenous. It is at this time that subtle renal parenchymal masses are best detected. The last phase, the excretory phase generally occurs 180 seconds after contrast administration. During this phase the renal calyces, pelvis, and ureters are opacified. Further delayed imaging may be necessary to ensure that all portions of the ureter have been opacified. [134]
Advanced protocols for contrast enhanced computerized tomography have been employed with the intention of gathering as much data as possible in examination of a renal mass. These protocols are directed toward differentiation of hyperdense cysts, complex cysts, and various types of solid renal masses i.e. oncocytomas, angiomyolipomas, and subtypes of renal cell carcinoma. These protocols often entail the identification of a region of interest within the mass in question, and then recording its density, in Hounsfield units, throughout the various phases of the study, which include the noncontrast phase, and the aforementioned contrast enhanced phases. Understanding the nature of multiphase CT is of critical importance in that enhancement is the most important factor in determining likelihood of malignancy. Furthermore, it appears that enhancement, which appears to be representative of the degree of angiogenesis, or vascularity within a tumor, also correlates to a degree with renal cell carcinoma tumor subtype [189]. CT enhancement is generally defined as an attenuation increase of at least 15-20 Hounsfield units (HU) from the corresponding noncontrast image. Lesions showing HU increases of 10-20 are not definitely categorized as enhancing masses due to a phenomenon known as cyst pseudoenhancement. As such, it is at times difficult to discern hypovascular lesions, such as papillary renal cell carcinoma from benign renal cysts. [135, 136]
Though not exclusively specific, certain types of renal masses tend to have relatively common features on multiphase computerized tomography. Angiomyolipomas often have fat components, which appear as low attenuation regions (generally negative Hounsfield units) seen best in the unenhanced phase. Histological subtypes of renal cell carcinoma generally are vascularized to different degrees, and may have characteristic enhancement "signatures" on multiphase contrast enhanced computerized tomography.

3.3.1 Advances in CT technology and technique

CT scanners are undergoing a continuing evolution. Newer generation scanners have larger numbers of detectors that exist in a variety of configurations. Additional detectors also allow for more helices to be generated. The purpose of the multiple detectors is the acquisition of isotropic data sets, allowing for reformatting in multiple planes with near equal resolution. The most recently produced scanners have 64-256 rows of detectors, which allow for rapid imaging and more precise imaging of smaller masses. This evolution may continue with even newer paradigms of detection that include an image plate detector. It is believed that this new advance may further improve imaging of very small structures, such as small renal masses and small renal blood vessels. Such technology may also result in less volume averaging and pixilation, factors that often limit imaging of complex cystic renal masses and small solid renal masses. [137]

In an attempt to limit radiation exposure, dual energy CT (DECT) has been extensively investigated. This technique involves retrospective removal of iodinated contrast from enhanced CT images, thus potentially eliminating need for the initial noncontrast scan via production of a virtual noncontrast scan. This technique has been applied more extensively to evaluation of urinary stones. However, as of most recent, a feasibility study with use of DECT equipped with a tin filter (for increased x-ray energy spectra separation) has shown improved sensitivity and specificity for discriminating cysts from enhancing masses in phantom models. [138] Early study of application of this technique in relation to renal masses has shown that single phase post contrast DECT, when reviewed in conjunction with the virtual noncontrast data set, had an accuracy of 94.6% in diagnosing malignant renal lesions, in comparison to 96% accuracy with use of multiphase CT examination. The reduction in radiation dose, with use of DECT, was 47%. [139] The full potential of this application will require further investigation.

Another new technique being introduced that may yet broaden the possibilities of tissue imaging with this modality is dynamic contrast enhanced CT, or perfusion CT. This evolving technique has the capability of assessing tissue perfusion in a noninvasive manner. [140, 141] The technique has been used for imaging both the brain and tumors. It may be particularly useful in evaluating tumors that are potentially treatable by antivascular therapies, by evaluating the efficacy of such therapies. As RCC is known for both angiogenesis and vascularity this technique may show promise. To date, perfusion CT has been used to show that highly vascularized metastatic renal tumors are associated with poorer prognosis. [142] However, a feasibility study suggested that perfusion CT provided significant data regarding tumor angiogenesis and histological subtype in primary renal tumors. [143] As such, it is possible that such prognostic capabilities may also be applicable to primary renal tumors.

3.3.2 Computerized tomography and differentiation of renal masses

On computerized tomography AML are generally of low Hounsfield unit attenuation value (-20 HU and less) in the unenhanced phase [37, 144], and have not been found to be associated with calcification as may be the case with renal cell carcinoma. [37, 145] Aneurysmal dilation is found in 50% of AMLs when they are visualized by angiography and can also suggest the diagnosis [37], but irregular vascularity can be seen in cases of renal cell carcinoma as well. However, fat poor angiomyolipomas may not show such features. In 14% of AMLs, fat cannot be identified with CT, presumably related to a reduced proportion of mature adipose tissue, and a definite diagnosis cannot be made. [37, 146] Milner et al noted that cases involving less than 25% fat/high power field on histologic analysis correlated with computerized tomographic findings where fat usually was not noted. [147] MRI However, newer generation CT scanners with improved spatial resolution are also useful for detection small amounts of gross fat not detected on MRI. [148] Otherwise, based on imaging, indeterminate cases are considered RCC until proven otherwise, which in turn may necessitate surgical intervention. Such lesions are only confirmed to be angiomyolipoma on final histopathological inspection.

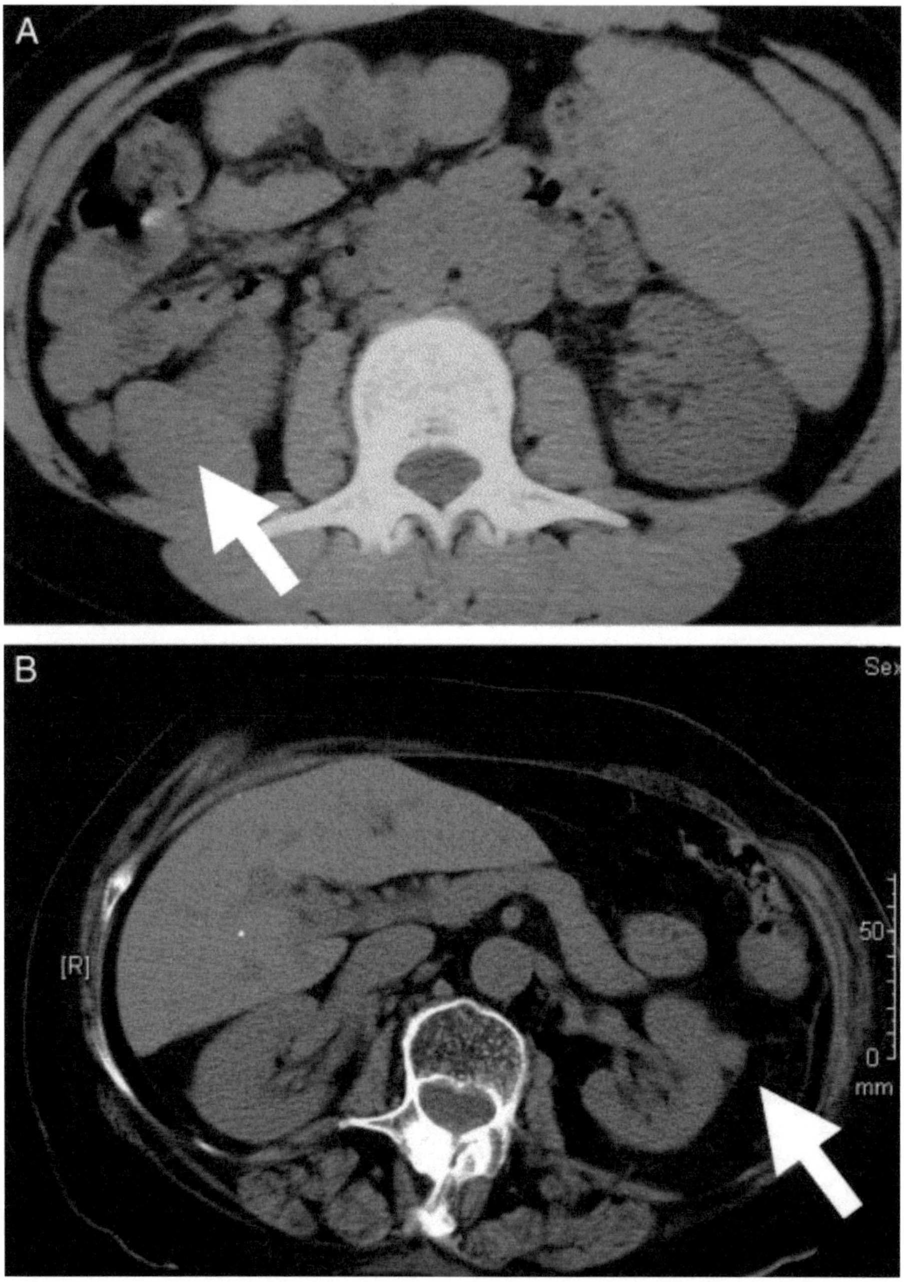

Fig. 4a and 4b. Nonenhanced CT shows hyperdense right (A) and isodense left (B) kidney lesions (arrow). Milner J, McNeil B, Alioto J,et al. (2006) fat poor angiomyolipoma: patient, computerized tomography and histological findings. *J Urol*; 176: 905-909

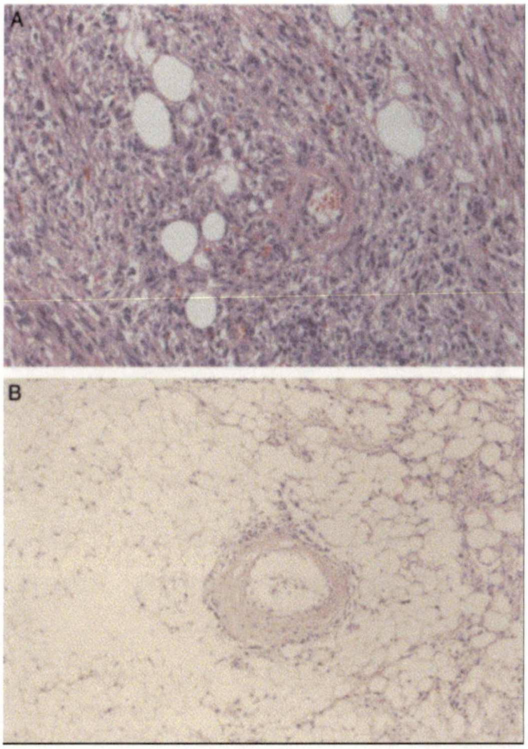

Fig. 5a and 5b. Fat poor lesion (A) with less than 25% fat and classic lesion (B) with greater than 75% fat and percent fat contents. H & E, reduced from x 40. Milner J, McNeil B, Alioto J,et al. (2006) fat poor angiomyolipoma: patient, computerized tomography and histological findings. *J Urol*; 176: 905-909

In a recent retrospective study of enhancing renal masses using dual phase (plain and nephrographic), masses (AML and non-AML) were evaluated with three different size (8-13 mm; 19-24 mm; and 30-35 mm) regions of interest placed (ROI) over the lowest attenuation value focus of the mass from images obtained in both phases. Different attenuation thresholds were studied and receiver operating characteristic (ROC) curves were derived. At attenuation threshld -10 HU and lower, with use of at least 19-24 mm ROI, on the unenhanced images, was found to be optimal for diagnosis of AML. At this threshold, misdiagnosis rate was 0.5%; at -15 HU threshold misdiagnosis rate was 0%. [149]

Renal oncocytoma is typically described to be a hypervascular, homogeneous mass that may contain a central stellate scar on computerized tomography (CT). However, extended experience has proved these findings to be unreliable and of poor predictive value [48, 49, 50, 51]. However, oncocytomas also appear to be quite vascular, and have a contrast uptake and drainage curve different from that of clear cell renal cell carcinoma.[12] In contrast study, both vascular uptake and washout should be closely examined. Though oncocytomas are considered histopathologically similar to chromophobe renal cell carcinoma, again, their enhance patterns seem to differ (see figure 2).

Enhancement patterns of renal tumors on computerized tomography have evolved to be a valuable non-invasive technique to help distinguish the different subtypes of renal cell carcinoma [150, 151]. Clear cell renal cell carcinomas are often quite vascularized, and often have high Hounsfield unit values in the early phases of the study immediately following contrast administration. Papillary renal cell carcinomas are relatively hypovascular and generally show mild enhancement during the study. Peak enhancement for papillary renal cell carcinomas may continue to increase during the latter corticomedullary and delayed phases of the study.[12]These different enhancement patterns can be seen in figure 1. Of interest, early investigation in a small number of tumors suggests that chromophobe RCC and oncocytoma may have different enhancement signatures; however, these findings require further investigation and corroboration.

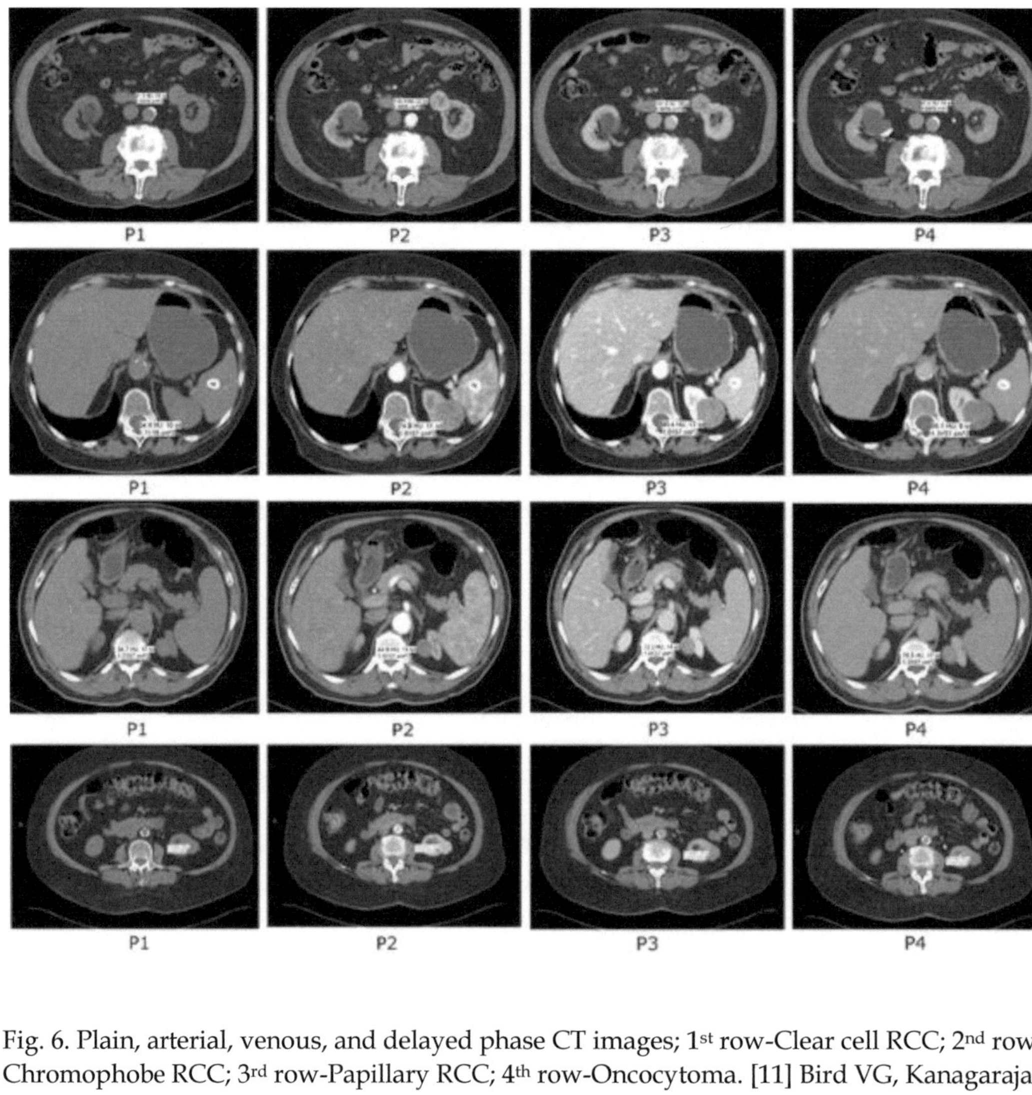

Fig. 6. Plain, arterial, venous, and delayed phase CT images; 1st row-Clear cell RCC; 2nd row-Chromophobe RCC; 3rd row-Papillary RCC; 4th row-Oncocytoma. [11] Bird VG, Kanagarajah P, Morillo G, et al. (2010). Differentiation of oncocytoma and renal cell carcinoma in small renal masses (<4 cm): the role of 4-phase computerized tomography. *World J Urol*; Aug. EPub.

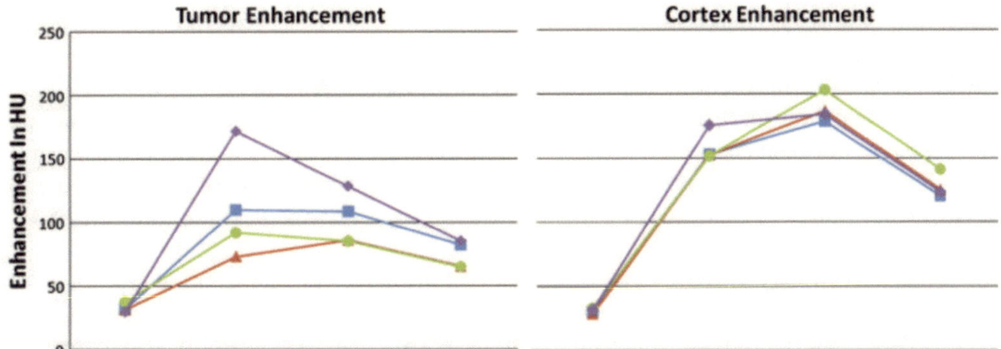

	P1	P2	P3	P4
Clear Cell	32.33	110.14	108.99	82.19
Papillary	31.47	73.14	85.8	65.3
Chromophobe	37.75	92.25	85.45	65.3
Oncocytoma	29.67	171.58	128.67	85.33

	C1	C2	C3	C4
Clear Cell	30.17	152.86	178.43	120.26
Papillary	28.67	152.24	186.33	125.19
Chromophobe	32.67	151.33	202.67	141
Oncocytoma	31.75	175	183.67	123

KEY: P1 tumor plain phase, P2 tumor arterial phase, P3 tumor venous phase, P4 tumor delayed phase C1 cortex plain phase, C2 cortex arterial phase, C3 cortex venous phase, C4 cortex delayed phase.

Fig. 7. Enhancement pattern of renal tumor and renal cortex on 4 phase CT [11]. Bird VG, Kanagarajah P, Morillo G, et al. (2010). Differentiation of oncocytoma and renal cell carcinoma in small renal masses (<4 cm): the role of 4-phase computerized tomography. World J Urol; Aug. EPub.)

3.4 Magnetic resonance imaging

The mechanism of magnetic resonance imaging essentially involves placement of the patient within a magnetic field, which results in the alignment of hydrogen protons in their body tissue. This alignment leads to the formation of a magnetic vector. This vector can be made to spin with application of a radiofrequency pulse. A wire (coil) outside the patient will then have a current induced within it by the magnetic force. The current emanating from the body tissue can then be measured. The magnitude of this current is related to the intensity of the pixel in the MR image. [152] MR information can be processed for creation of direct multiplanar images i.e. transverse, sagittal, and coronal (CT data is acquired in the transverse plane). Due to its nature, MR may yield particularly unique information regarding blood flow and fluid composition, which is useful in a variety of circumstances, namely the identification of fluid and blood in renal cysts and tumor associated renal vein/inferior vena cava thrombus. MR of the kidneys is generally performed on 1.5 or 3 Tesla magnets. The standard sequences used for MR evaluation of a renal mass include T1 weighted imaging (in and out of phase sequences), T2 weighted images in two planes, fat suppressed T1 weighted gradient echo acquisition before and after contrast administration at multiple time points, including arterialcorticomedullary, nephrographic, and urographic phases. [148] Individual institutions also often have slight modifications of this protocol.

Acquired MR data can be further analyzed with analysis of subtraction images (subtracting precontrast image from post contrast images). This technique aids in detection of enhancement. In such analyses, areas of high signal appear only in areas of enhancement. [148] In a comparison, for identification of renal malignancy subtraction imaging was more sensitive (99%) when compared to quantitative (quantitative enhancement ratio calculation) evaluation (95%). [153]

Contraindications to performance of MRI include those with pacemakers, ferromagnetic intracranial aneurysm clips, cochlear implants, metallic ocular foreign bodies and some particular makes of older prosthetic heart valves. For MR imaging, breath holding is necessary for proper data acquisition. New generation scanners, with more rapid acquisition times, have allowed for much more practical and reasonable patient breath-holding, however, many a patient has complained about the amount time spent in the confined space of an MR scanner. Open MR scanners are available; however, image quality may be a concern.

For contrast-enhanced MRI, gadolinium, a paramagnetic lanthanide metal, used in conjunction with chelates, acts as the contrast agent. This contrast agent is quite different from iodine based contrast material used in plain film radiography and computerized tomography. It is not specifically nephrotoxic. [154] Gadolinium-based MR contrast agents are associated with less allergic reactions that iodinated contrast agents. [155] It is generally safe for those with a history of allergic reaction to iodinated contrast material. [155, 156, 157] This makes MR imaging attractive for use in the assessment of renal disorders in children, women of childbearing age, and those with renal allografts. [158]

For some time gadolinium enhanced MRI had been an imaging preference for patients with renal insufficiency. However, the use of gadolinium based contrast agents in patients with limited renal function has become a concern. In 1997, a condition, later termed nephrogenic systemic fibrosis (NSF), was noted to occur in a small number of patients undergoing MRI with gadolinium based contrast agents. The condition was first noted in patients with renal failure, and involves progressive fibrosis of the skin and other body tissues. This issue was recently extensively reviewed , delineating the risks of gadolinium exposure in patients with glomerular filtration rate (GFR) less than 30 mL/min. The risk of NSF appears to be very low in patients with higher GFR. [159]

Contrast of different body tissue on MR examination differs from that of CT. Important factors include proton density, T1 and T2 and magnetic susceptibility, and flow. In MR terminology, T1 is a measure of how quickly a tissue can become magnetized and T2 relates to how quickly a given body tissue loses it magnetization. MR protocols for renal masses vary slightly, but essentially include precontrast T1 and T2 fast spin echo sequences, where elements of assessment include discerning the presence of fat (bright T1 signal), hemorrhage (bright T1 signal), and cystic lesions (bright T2 signal). [117] Axial acquisition is preferred as comparison to CT images is often done. Images acquired in the axial plane generally yield the best vascular images as well. Similar techniques are used during the precontrast and contrast -enhanced portions of the exam to allow for proper comparison. Other techniques, such as frequency-selective fat-suppression techniques (FATSAT) or chemical shift (in- and out-of phase) help distinguish the presence of fat from that of hemorrhage in a renal lesion. Specific techniques are also used to assess for flow defects within the renal vein and inferior vena cava. Cardiac synchronized sequence can be used if initial techniques are inconclusive in cases of determination of the presence of renal vein/inferior vena cava thrombus (thrombus results in persistent filling defect over the entire cardiac cycle). [160]

On MR imaging, enhancement is measured in terms of signal intensity. Similar to CT, motion artifact, volume averaging, and fluctuations in signal intensity may result in pseudoenhancement. For a 0.1 mmol/kg contrast dose on a 1.5 T MR scanner 15% enhancement over the baseline precontrast signal has been considered 'significant" enhancement, though it is important to understand that this value may not be applicable to other scanners, field strengths, and imaging techniques. [160]

MRI is useful for differentiation of solid renal masses and cysts. Due to reasons related to cost and availability, urologic evaluations with use of MRI are generally reserved for patients with iodinated contrast toxicity, masses still regarded as indeterminate on CT scan, and cases where there is adequate suspicion for renal vein/inferior vena cava thrombus. MR imaging is considered excellent for vascular structures and the liver, and as such is considered both necessary and useful in cases where the possible presence of renal vein and inferior vena cava tumor associated thrombus needs to be assessed. Various MR techniques may be used to assess for fat within renal tumors, however, as is the case with CT, fat poor angiomyolipomas exist and thus make specific radiologic diagnosis of this entity not always certain.

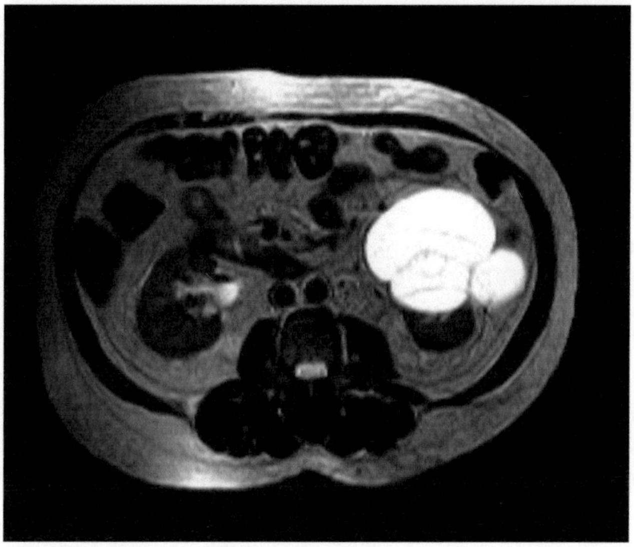

Fig. 8. In this patient with renal insufficiency (serum creatinine 3.5 ng/dl) T2 weighted images of an unenhanced MRI show a complex left renal lesion to be only cystic in nature, and without solid elements. (Courtesy of author)

As has been done with CT scanning, attempts have been made to use differential intensity of signal enhancement with MR imaging in order to aid differentiation of benign versus malignant masses, namely differentiating benign oncocytomas from malignant renal cell carcinomas. Recent investigations protocols focus on reliable differentiation of these two groups of tumors.

Due to concerns of repeated exposure to ionizing radiation, MR may be preferable CT for active surveillance in patient with renal mass who are either poor candidates for surgery or have otherwise elected this option.

3.4.1 Advances in magnetic resonance technology and technique

Some of the latest advances in MR include use of diffusion weighted imaging, which quantifies the thermally induced motion of water molecules (Brownian motion) in tissues. Restriction of water motion or its diffusion is qualitatively or quantitatively evaluated by means of an apparent diffusion coefficient (ADC) measure. [148] This technique appears quite useful in that DWI does not require gadolinium administration and appears to provide information regarding tumor microenvironment. Malignant masses appear to have lower ADC than benign ones. This is thought to be due to the high cellularity/complex architecture of neoplastic lesions. [161, 162] It has been further noted that higher Fuhrman grade renal cell carcinomas have lower ADC than lower grade lesions. [163]. Diffusion weighted imaging has also been studied in differentiation of solid and cystic lesions. Again, solid lesions have very low ADC, whereas cysts have higher ADC, Bosniak type 1 cysts had the highest ADC. [164]

3.4.2 Magnetic resonance imaging and differentiation of renal masses

A strength of MRI relates to its characterization of fluid filled entities. It is thus not only accurate in terms of identification of simple renal cysts, but is also quite useful in characterization of cystic renal masses, even in cases where limited renal function or other contraindication preclude gadolinium administration. In a study using Bosniak criteria for evaluation of cystic lesions, 10% of cases were upstaged due to features detected on MRI. MRI appears to be quite useful in detecting the presence, thickness, and enhancement of septa. [18, 165]

Fat-suppressed images on MRI may be helpful in difficult cases or when CT is contraindicated for other reasons. MRI is useful in detection of both macroscopic and microscopic fat in angiomyolipomas. Macroscopic fat can be seen on T1 weighted out of phase sequence and often shows a black outline around the lesion that has been termed the "india ink artifact". In one study this artifact was seen in 100% of AML and 4% non-AML lesions [166]. Microscopic fat not seen on CT can also be detected with chemical shift (in and out of phase) imaging. In these cases, signal loss from the in-phase to opposed-phase images may increase diagnostic confidence for fat poor angiomyolipomas. However, one must bear in mind that clear cell type renal cell carcinoma may contain intracytoplasmic lipid glycogen/lipid that may also manifest as a similar signal loss. [148]

In a recent study, the value of MR T2 weighted imaging was evaluated for diagnosis of AML. The investigators analyzed a group of patients who had undergone CT for enhancing mass with no visible fat. Signal intensity and signal intensity ratio were measured. The signal intensity ratios for AML and non-AML were compared and subjected to receiver operating characteristic (ROC) analysis. Results demonstrated significantly lower signal intensity ratio values for AML. Though promising, the study only contained a small number of angiomyolipomas and will require further investigation. [167]

Characteristic findings for oncocytoma on MRI include well-defined capsule, central stellate scar, and distinctive intensities on T1 and T2 images, all of which can suggest the diagnosis but cannot be considered definitive. [168] MR comparison of chromophobe renal cell carcinoma and oncocytoma shows no significant differences. MR study of enhancement patterns of the clear cell, papillary, and chromophobe forms of renal cell carcinoma has been performed, showing some distinctive enhancement patterns for each of the three subtypes, however, no comparison was made to oncocytoma, the benign tumor that is of critical consideration in this differential diagnosis. [94]

Studies also have shown that papillary RCCs are hypointense on T2-weighted imaging, likely due to old blood products, whereas clear cell RCCs tend to be T2 iso- to hyperintense. Though enhancing renal masses are reliably detected on MRI, renal cell tumor subtyping has not been as extensively investigated in a manner similar to that of CT.

4. Nuclear imaging

The general premise of nuclear imaging involves the administration of radionuclide labeled molecules for a specific purpose for assessment of both physiologic and anatomic details that is not obtainable with other radiologic imaging modalities. Information is gathered by a gamma scintillation camera, which now commonly rotate in a number of directions. Studies more functional in nature may show limited anatomic detail, but newer technologies and complex programming have allowed for more advanced integration of physiologic process/function and related anatomy. Radiation exposure with these techniques is minimal, and valuable functional information, and more recently, functional/anatomic information, may be obtained. Nuclear imaging studies have been employed widely throughout medical specialties and offer great potential as further molecular and physiologic aspects of a number of disease processes are better understood.

Nuclear imaging is more often used to assess extent of disease rather than the specific characteristics of primary renal tumor. However, the possibilities employing techniques using this modality are far reaching. Ready procurement of the needed radionuclide and its bound molecule can at times limit availability of this imaging modality.

4.1 Advances in nuclear imaging technique and technology

Research involving potentiating the application of nuclear medicine in specific tumor identification can be seen in the development of radiolabelled aptamers. The premise involves the production of specific receptor binding molecules based on defined nucleic acid sequences that are capable of recognizing a wide array of target molecules. Aptamers can now be readily produced and are stable. These molecules are generally small, as small as 5-10 kDa, and readily penetrate into tumors. Current efforts focus on manipulating the molecular weight of these molecules to achieve optimal balance between low immunogenicity, good tumor penetration/uptake, and renal clearance. [169]

4.2 Nuclear imaging and differentiation of renal masses

The nuclear agent technetium sestamibi is evidently retained in mitochondria, with reported increased uptake in oncocytomas compared with RCC, AML, and renal cysts. The biologic rationale for nuclear scanning is therefore strong, but these results have not been confirmed, and their clinical role or utility has not been developed. [170]

As aforementioned, ultrasonography, computerized tomography, and magnetic resonance imaging are all commonly used in the evaluation and diagnosis of renal masses. However, a common criticism is that they mostly provide a morphometric analysis, are indeed sensitive, but not very specific. Fluorine-18 fluorodeoxyglucose positron emission tomography (F-18 FDG PET) has been used in diagnosis, differential diagnosis, staging, follow-up, therapy planning, and prognostication in a number of malignancies. [171, 172, 173, 174]. The premise of this imaging technique is that malignant tissues have a higher uptake of FDG than do surrounding normal tissues. This is due to higher levels of glucose transporter proteins and glucose transfer in cancer cells. [175, 176]. PET/CT studies are carried out using a PET/CT integrated scanner. The clinical role of F-18 FDG PET in evaluation of renal masses has yet to be determined, partly because of the physiological excretion of FDG through the kidneys, which makes it difficult to visualize the structures and tumors against the high background of FDG. Different studies to date have reported a wide range of sensitivities for F-18 FDG

PET in this role, with sensitivities ranging from 40-94%. [177, 178]. As of most recent, a prospective study done to further evaluate the role of PET/CT in this setting concluded that a positive PET/CT may indicate the presence of renal cell carcinoma, but that a negative study did not rule it out. The authors noted that higher Furman grade and larger tumor sized increased detection of renal cell carcinoma by PET/CT. [179] The authors also noted a false positive result associated with oncocytoma. Previous studies also noted that oncocytomas can yield false positive results on F-18 FDG-PET/CT [21,41]. [180, 181] In a study by Goldberg et al. [182], patients with indeterminate renal cysts were examined and F-18 FDG-PET/CT accurately detected 10 cysts as benign with no false positive results.

To date this modality appears to only have a limited role in evaluation of renal tumor but may be useful as an adjunct study where more standard imaging modalities only yield equivocal results. PET scanning may gain a larger role in staging rather than with evaluation of primary tumors

5. Conclusion

Imaging plays a critical role in the evaluation of renal masses. It is most often the deciding factor in determining whether invasive intervention is necessary. As active surveillance has become an option for some patients, the importance of imaging is only heightened. In addition to differentiation of benign and malignant tumors, better imaging is needed for proper noninvasive identification of those neoplasms of low versus higher malignant potential. At the current time, a large body of research now exists relating to their more specific characterization. Multiphase CT characterization of renal masses has been the foundation of this research, though certainly other modalities, notably contrast enhanced ultrasound, dual energy CT, and diffusion weighted MRI also hold promise. New imaging techniques appear to have improved preoperative identification of angiomyolipoma. Renal oncocytomas have eluded reliable preoperative imaging, but new CT data demonstrates that further investigation into the details of these tumors may also make them identifiable preoperatively. As these tumors relate closely to chromophobe renal cell carcinoma, further molecular studies and characterization of these lesions will likely aid in their proper identification and classification. Use of CT imaging, through exploitation of the vascular nature of renal tumors, has opened the door and demonstrated that specific characterization of renal masses by noninvasive imaging is feasible and should be further studied. Despite its advantages in image resolution and quality, research relating to modification of CT protocols so as to limit exposure to ionizing radiation is also of great importance. The new paradigm of PET/CT imaging is in its infancy and may yet show future promise in terms of providing physiopathologic data in addition to anatomic data. Though any one imaging modality has not yet been demonstrated to be entirely reliable for specific and highly reliable characterization of renal masses, in many cases it appears that a combination of these studies may increase diagnostic certainty, or at a minimum, better direct clinicians in identification of patients who may specifically benefit from percutaneous biopsy. Future directions in the study of renal imaging include further minimizing exposure to ionizing radiation and contrast media related toxicity; further manipulation of advanced imaging protocols to differentiate tissue related differences in renal tumors; and further integration of studies that will yield more specific anatomic and physiopathologic information.

6. References

[1] Jemal A, Siegel R, Xu J, et al. (2010). Cancer Statistics, 2010. *CA Cancer J Clin*; 60: 277-300.

[2] Kirkali Z, Obek C. (2003). Clinical aspects of renal cell carcinoma. *EAU Update Ser*; 1: 189–96.

[3] Lipworth L, Tarone RE, McLaughlin JK. (2006). The epidemiology of renal cell carcinoma. *J Urol*. Dec;176(6 Pt 1): 2353–2358.

[4] Campbell SC, Novick AC, Belldegrun A, et al. (2009). Guideline for management of T1 renal mass. *J Urol*; 182: 1271-1279.

[5] Kutikov A, Fossett LK and Ramchandani P, et al. (2008). Incidence of benign pathologic findings at partial nephrectomy for solitary renal mass presumed to be renal cell carcinoma on preoperative imaging. *BJU Int*; 68 p. 737-742.

[6] Snyder ME, Bach A, Kattan MW, et al. (2006). Incidence of benign lesions for clinically localized renal masses smaller than 7 cm in radiological diameter: influence of sex. *J Urol*; 176, p. 2391-2395.

[7] Pahernik S, Ziegler S, Roos F, et al. (2007). Small renal tumors: correlation of clinical and pathological features with tumor size, *J Urol*; 178 p. 414-417.

[8] Remzi M, Ozsoy M, Klingler HC, et al. (2006). Are small renal tumors harmless? Analysis of histopathological features according to tumors 4 cm or less in diameter. *J Urol*; 176 p. 896-899.

[9] Tsivian M, Mouraviev V, Albala DM, et al. (2011). Clinical predictors of renal mass pathological features. *BJU Int*; Mar;107(5):735-40.

[10] Volpe A. Cadeddu JA, Cestari A, et al. (2011). Contemporary management of small renal masses. *Eur Urol*. Jun 1. [Epub ahead of print].

[11] Sheir KZ, El-Azab M, Mosbah A, et al. (2005). Differentiation of renal cell carcinoma subtypes by multislice computerized tomography. *J Urol*; 174(2):451–455.

[12] Kim JK, Kim TK, Ahn HJ, et al. (2002). Differentiation of subtypes of renal cell carcinoma on helical CT scans. *AJR Am J Roentgenol*; 178(6):1499–1506.

[13] Bird VG, Kanagarajah P, Morillo G, et al. (2010). Differentiation of oncocytoma and renal cell carcinoma in small renal masses (<4 cm): the role of 4-phase computerized tomography. *World J Urol*; Aug. EPub.

[14] Park SY, Jeon SS, Lee Sy, et al. (2011). Incidence and predictive factors of benign renal lesions in Korean patients with preoperative imaging diagnoses of renal cell carcinoma. *J Korean Med Sci*; 26: 360-364.

[15] Mason RJ, Abdolell M, and Rendon RA. (2010). Tumour location as a predictor of benign disease in the management of renal masses. *CUAJ*; 4: 414-418.

[16] Lane BR, Babineau D, Kattan, et al. (2007). A preoperative prognostic nomogram for solid enhancing renal tumours 7 cm or less amenable to partial nephrectomy. *J Urol*; 178: 429-444.

[17] Bosniak MA. (1986). The current radiological approach to renal cysts. *Radiology*; (158): 1–10.

[18] Israel GM, Hindman N, and Bosniak MA. (2004). Comparison of CT and MRI in the evaluation of cystic renal masses. *Radiology*; (231):365–371.

[19] Israel GM and Bosniak MA. (2005). An update of the Bosniak renal cyst classification system. *Urology*; 66 (3): 484-488.

[20] Curry NS, Cochran ST, and Bissada NK. (2000). Cystic renal masses accurate Bosniak classification requires adequate renal CT. *AJR Am J Roentgenol*; (175): 339–342.

[21] Koga S, Nishikido M, Inuzuka S, et al. (2000). An evaluation of Bosniak's radiological classification of cystic renal masses. *BJU Int;* (86): 607–609.

[22] Levy P, Helenon O, Merran S, et al. (1999). Cystic tumors of the kidney in adults radio-histopathologic correlations. *J Radiol;* (80): 121–133.

[23] Israel GM and Bosniak MA. (2003). Follow-up CT studies for moderately complex cystic renal masses (Bosniak category IIF). *AJR Am J Roentgenol;* (181): 627–633.

[24] Israel GM and Bosniak MA. (2003). Calcification in cystic renal masses is it important in diagnosis?, *Radiology;* (226): 47–52.

[25] Siegel CL, Middleton WD, Teefey SA, et al. (1996). Angiomyolipoma and renal cell carcinoma: US differentiation. *Radiology;* 198:789-793.

[26] Renshaw AA, Granter SR, and Cibas ES. (1997). Fine-needle aspiration of the adult kidney. *Cancer;* (81): 71–88.

[27] Dechet CB, Zincke H, Sebo TJ, et al. (2003). Prospective analysis of computerized tomography and needle biopsy with permanent sectioning to determine the nature of solid renal masses in adults. *J Urol;* (169): 71–74.

[28] Bosniak MA. (2003). Should we biopsy complex cystic renal masses (Bosniak category III)?, *AJR Am J Roentgenol;* (181): 1425–1426.

[29] Hayakawa M, Hatano T, Tsuji A, et al. (1996). Patients with renal cysts associated with renal cell carcinoma and the clinical implications of cyst puncture a study of 223 cases. *Urology;* (47): 643–646.

[30] Horwitz CA, Manivel JC, Inampudi S, et al. (1994). Diagnostic difficulties in the interpretation of needle aspiration material from large renal cysts. *Diag Cytopathol;* (11): 380–383.

[31] Tamboli P, Ro JY, Amin MB, et al. (2000). Benign tumors and tumor-like lesions of the adult kidney, part II: Benign mesenchymal and mixed neoplasms, and tumor-like lesions. *Adv Anat Pathol;* 7:47-66.

[32] Nelson CP, Sanda MG. (2002). Contemporary diagnosis and management of renal angiomyolipoma. *J Urol;* 168:1315-1325.

[33] Eble JN. Angiomyolipoma of kidney. (1998). *Semin Diagn Pathol;* 15:21-40.

[34] Neumann HP, Schwarzkopf G, Hensk EP. (1998). Renal angiomyolipomas, cysts, and cancer in tuberous sclerosis complex. *Semin Pediatr Neurol;* 5:269-275.

[35] Lendvay TS, Marshall FF. (2003). The tuberous sclerosis complex and its highly variable manifestations. *J Urol;* 169:1635-1642.

[36] Oesterling JE, Fishman EK, Goldman SM, et al. (1986). The management of renal angiomyolipoma. *J Urol;* 135:1121-1124.

[37] Lemaitre L, Robert Y, Dubrulle F, et al. (1995). Renal angiomyolipoma: Growth followed up with CR and/or US. *Radiology;* 197:598-602.

[38] Turker I, Tunc M, Kilicaslan I, et al. (2000). Lymph nodal involvement by renal angiomyolipoma. *Int J Urol;* 7:386-389.

[39] Gogus C, Safak M, Erekul S, et al. (2001). Angiomyolipoma of the kidney with lymph node involvement in a 17-year-old female mimicking renal cell carcinoma: A cell report. *Int Urol Nephrol;* 33:617-618.

[40] Christiano AP, Yang X, Gerber GS, et al. (1999). Malignant transformation of renal angiomyolipoma. *J Urol;* 161:1900-1901.

[41] Ferry JA, Malt RA, Young RH. (1991). Renal angiomyolipoma with sarcomatous transformation and pulmonary metastases. *Am J Surg Pathol;* 15:1083-1088.

[42] Lieber MM, Hosaka Y, Tsukamoto T: (1987). Renal oncocytoma. *World J Urol;* 5:71-79.

[43] Gill IS, Kamoi K, Aron M, et al: (2010) 800 laparoscopic partial nephrectomies: a single surgeon series. *J Urol; 183: 34-41.*

[44] Amin MB, Crotty TB, Tickoo SK, et al. (1997b). Renal oncocytoma: A reappraisal of morphologic features with clinicopathologic findings in 80 cases. *Am J Surg Pathol;* 21:1-12.

[45] Kuroda N, Toi M, Hiroi M, et al. (2003d). Review of renal oncocytoma with focus on clinical and pathobiological aspects. *Histol Histopathol;* 18:935-942.

[46] Perez-Ordonez B, Hamed G, Campbell S, et al. (1997). Renal oncocytoma: A clinicopathological study of 70 cases. *Am J Surg Pathol;* 21:871-883.

[47] Israel GM and Silverman SG: (2011). The incidental renal mass. *Radiol Clin North Am;* 49: 369-383.

[48] Levine E, Huntrakoon M: (1983). Computed tomography of renal oncocytoma. *AJR Am J Roentgenol;* 141:741-746.

[49] Davidson AJ, Hayes WS, Hartman DS, et al. (1993). Renal oncocytoma and carcinoma: Failure of differentiation with CT imaging. *Radiology;* 183:693-696.

[50] Zisman A, Patard JJ, Raz O, et al. (2010) sex, age, and surgeon decision on nephron-sparing surgery are independent predictors of renal masses with benign histologic findings-a multicenter survey. *Urology*: 76: 541-546.

[51] Licht MR. (1995). Renal adenoma and oncocytoma. *Semin Urol Oncol;* 13:262-266.

[52] Farrow GM: Diseases of the kidney. In Murphy WM, ed: Urological Pathology, 2nd ed. Philadelphia, WB Saunders, 1997:464-470.

[53] Renshaw AA: Subclassification of renal cell neoplasms: (2002). An update for the practicing pathologist. *Histopathology;* 41:283-300.

[54] Trpkov K, Yilmaz A, Uzer D, et al. Renal oncocytomas revisited: a clinicopatholigic study of 109 cases with emphasis on problematic diagnostic features. (2010). *Histopathology;* 57: 893-906.

[55] Minor LD, Picken MM, Campbell SC, et al. Benign renal tumors. (2003). AUA Update; 22:170-175.

[56] Linehan WM, Walther MM, Zbar B. (2003). The genetic basis of cancer of the kidney. *J Urol;* 170:2163-2172.

[57] Pavlovich CP, Grubb RL, Hurley K, et al. (2005). Evaluation and management of renal tumors in the Birt-Hogg-Dubé syndrome. *J Urol;* 173:1482-1486.

[58] Dechet CB, Bostwick DG, Blute Ml, et al. (1999). Renal oncocytomas: multifocality, bilateralism, metachronous tumor development, and co-existent renal cell carcinoma. *J Urol*: 162: 40-42.

[59] Licht MR, Novick AC, Tubbs RR, et al. (1993). Renal oncocytomas: clinical and biological correlates. *J Urol;* 150: 1380-1383.

[60] Davis CJ, Mostofi FK, Sesterhenn IA, et al. (1991). Renal oncocytomas. Clinicopathologic study of 166 patients. *J Urogenital Pathol;* 1: 41-52.

[61] Romis L, Cindolo L, Patard JJ, et al. (2004). Frequency, clinical presentation and evolution of renal oncocytomas: multicentric experience from a European database. *Eur Urol;* 45: 53-57.

[62] Gudbjartsson T, Hardarson S, Petursdottir V, et al. (2005). Renal oncocytomas: a clinicopathologic analysis of 45 consecutive cases. *BJU Int;* 96: 1275-1279.

[63] Neuzillet Y Lechevallier E, Andre M, et al. (2005). Follow-up of renal oncocytomas diagnosed by percutaneous tumor biopsy. *Urology*; 66: 1181-1185.

[64] Fan YH, Chang YH, Huang WJS, et al. (2008). Renal oncocytomas: clinical experience of Taipei Veterans general hospital. *J Chin Med Assoc*; 71; 254-258.

[65] Chao DH, Zisman A, Pantuck AJ, et al. (2002a). Changing concepts in the management of renal oncocytoma. *Urology*; 59:635-642.

[66] Landis SH, Murray T, Bolden S, Wingo PA. Cancer statistics: 1999. (1999). *CA Cancer J Clin*; 49:8-31.

[67] Pantuck AJ, Zisman A, Belldegrun AS. (2001b). The changing natural history of renal cell carcinoma. *J Urol*; 166:1611-1623.

[68] Chow WH, Devesa SS, Warren JL, et al. (1999). Rising incidence of renal cell cancer in the United States. *JAMA*; 281:1628-1631.

[69] Parsons JK, Schoenberg MS, Carter HB. (2001). Incidental renal tumors: Casting doubt on the efficacy of early intervention. *Urology*; 57:1013-1015.

[70] Raz O, Mendlovic, Leibovici D, et al. (2007). The prevalence of malignancy in renal satellite lesions and its surgical implication during nephron sparing surgery. *J Urol*; 178: 1892-1895.

[71] Campbell SC, Fichter J, Novick AC, et al: (1996a). Intraoperative evaluation of renal cell carcinoma: A prospective study of the roles of ultrasonography and histopathological frozen sections. *J Urol*; 155:1191-1195.

[72] Klatte T, Wunderlich H, Patard JJ, et al. Clinicopathologic features and prognosis of synchronous bilateral renal cell carcinoma: an international multicenter experience. (2007). *BJU Int*; 100: 21-25.

[73] Farrow GM: Diseases of the kidney. In Murphy WM, ed: Urological Pathology, 2nd ed. Philadelphia, WB Saunders, 1997:464-470.

[74] Mukamel E, Konichezky M, Engelstein D, et al. (1988). Incidental small renal tumors accompanying clinically overt renal cell carcinoma. *J Urol*; 140:22-24.

[75] Richstone L, Scherr D, Reuter VR, et al. (2004). Multifocal renal cortical tumors: Frequency, associated clinicopathological features and impact on survival. *J Urol*; 171:615-620.

[76] Störkel S. Classification of renal cancer: Correlation of morphology and cytogenetics. In Vogelzang NJ, Scardino PT, Shipley WU, Coffey DS, eds: Comprehensive Textbook of Genitourinary Oncology, 2nd ed. Baltimore, Williams & Wilkins, 1996:179-186.

[77] Oyasu R. Renal cancer: (1998). Histologic classification update. *Int J Clin Oncol*; 3:125-133.

[78] Pantuck AJ, Zisman A, Belldegrun A. (2001a) Biology of renal cell carcinoma: Changing concepts in classification and staging. *Semin Urol Oncol*; 19:72-79.

[79] Lindgren D, Bostrom AK, Nilsson K, et al. (2011). Isolation and characterization of progenitor-like cells from human renal proximal tubules. Am J Pathol; 178: 828-837.

[80] Rabbani F, Hakimian P, Reuter V, et al. (2004). Renal vein or inferior vena caval extension in patients with renal cortical tumors: Impact of tumor histology. *J Urol*; 171:1057-1061.

[81] Davis CJ, Mostofi FK, Sesterhenn IA. Renal medullary carcinoma: (1995). The seventh sickle cell nephropathy. *Am J Surg Pathol*; 19:1-11.

[82] Herts BR, Baker ME. (1995). The current role of percutaneous biopsy in the evaluation of renal masses. *Semin Urol Oncol*; 13:254-261.

[83] Schatz SM, Lieber MM. (2003). Update on oncocytoma. *Curr Urol Rep;* 4:30-35.

[84] Silver DA, Morash C, Brenner P, et al. (1997). Pathologic findings at the time of nephrectomy for renal masses. *Ann Surg Oncol;* 4:570-574.

[85] Leveridge MJ, Finelli A, Kachura JR, et al: (2011) Outcomes of small renal mass needle core biopsy, nondiagnostic percutaneous biopsy, and the role of repeat biopsy. *Eur Urol;* June; Epub ahead of print.

[86] Hopper KD, and Yakes WF. (1990). The posterior intercostal approach for percutaneous renal procedures: Risk of puncturing the lung, spleen, and liver as determined by CT. *AJR Am J Roentgenol;* 154:115-117.

[87] Vassiliades VG, Bernardino ME. (1991). Percutaneous renal and adrenal biopsies. *Cardiovasc Intervent Radiol;* 14:50-54.

[88] Corica FA, Iczkowski KA, Cheng L, et al. (1999). Cystic renal cell carcinoma is cured by resection: A study of 24 cases with long-term follow-up. *J Urol;* 161:408-411.

[89] Koga S, Nishikido M, Hayashi T, et al. (2000). Outcome of surgery in cystic renal cell carcinoma. *J Urol;* 56:67-70.

[90] Nassir A, Jollimore J, Gupta R, et al. (2002). Multilocular cystic renal cell carcinoma: A series of 12 cases and review of the literature. *Adult Urol;* 60:421-427.

[91] Imura J, Ichikawa K, Takeda J, et al. (2004). Multilocular cystic renal cell carcinoma: A clinicopathological, immuno- and lectin histochemical study of nine cases. *APMIS;* 112:183-191.

[92] Skinner DG, Pfister RF, Colvin R. (1972). Extension of renal cell carcinoma into the vena cava: The rationale for aggressive surgical management. *J Urol;* 107:711-716.

[93] Schefft P, Novick AC, Straffon RA, et al. (1978). Surgery for renal cell carcinoma extending into the inferior vena cava. *J Urol;* 120:28-31.

[94] Sun MR, Ngo L, Genega EM, et al. (2009). Renal cell carcinoma: dynamic contrast-enhanced MR imaging for differentiation of tumor subtypes—correlation with pathologic findings. *Radiology,* 250:793–802.

[95] Pedrosa I, Chou MT, Ngo L, et al. (2008). MR classification of renal masses with pathologic correlation. *Eur Radiol,* 18:365–375.

[96] Herts BR, Coll DM, Novick AC, et al. (2002). Enhancement characteristics of papillary renal neoplasms revealed on triphasic helical CT of the kidneys. *AJR Am J Roentgenol,* 178:367–372.

[97] Herts BR. The current status of CT urography. (2002). *Crit Rev Comput Tomogr;* 43: 219-241.

[98] McTavish JD, Jinzaki M, Zou KH, et al. (2002). Multi-detector row CT urography: comparison of strategies for depicting the normal urinary collecting system. *Radiology;* 225: 783-790.

[99] Caoili EM, Cohan RH, Korobkin M, et al. (2002). Urinary tract abnormalities: initial experience with multi-detector row CT urography. *Radiolgy;* 222: 353-360.

[100] Noroozian M, Cohan RH, Caoili EM, et al. (2004). Multislice CT Urography: state of the art. *BJR* 77: S74-S86.

[101] Zilberman DE, Tsivian M, Lipkin ME, et al. (2011). Low dose computerized tomography for detection of urolithiasis--its effectiveness in the setting of the urology clinic. *J Urol.* Mar;185(3):910-4. Epub 2011 Jan 15.

[102] Morris TW. (1993). The physiologic effects of nonionic contrast media on the heart. *Invest Radiol;* 28: S44-S46.

[103] Stormorken H, Skalpe IO, and Testart MC. (1986). Effects of various contrast media on coagulation, fibrinolysis, and platelet function: an in vitro and in vivo study. *Invest Radiol*; 21: 348-354.

[104] Porter GA: Effects of contrast agents on renal function. (1993). *Invest Radiol*; 28 S1-S5.

[105] Porter GA: contrast media-associated nephrotoxicity. (1993). Recognition and management. *Invest Radiol*; 28: S11-S18.

[106] Mudge GH. (1980). Nephrotoxicity of Urographic Radiocontrast Drugs. *Kidney Int*; 18: 540-552.

[107] Barrett BJ and Carlisle EJ. (1993) Meta-analysis of the relative nephrotoxicity of high and low osmolality iodinated contrast media. *Radiology*; 188: 171.

[108] Thompsen HS and Morcos SK. (1999). Contrast media and metformin: guideline to diminish the risk of lactic acidosis in noninsulin dependent diabetics after administration of contrast agents. *Eur Radiol*; 9: 738-740.

[109] Katayama H, Yamaguchi K, Kozuka t, et al. (1990). Adverse reactions to ionic and nonionic contrast media. *Radiology*; 175: 621-628.

[110] Caro JJ, Trindade E, and McGregor M. (1991). The risks of death and of severe nonfatal reactions with high vs low-osmolality contrast media: A meta-analysis. *AJR Am J Roentgenol*; 156: 825-832.

[111] Greenberger PA and Patterson R. (1991). The prevention of immediate generalized reactions to radiocontrast media in high-risk patients. *J Allergy Clin Immunol*; 87: 867-872.

[112] Lasser EC, Berry CC, Mishkin MM, et al. (1994). Pretreatment with corticosteroids to prevent adverse reactions to nonionic contrast media. *AJR Am J Roentgenol*; 162: 523-526.

[113] Sears CL, Ward JF, Sears ST, et al. (2002). Prospective comparison of computerized tomography and excretory urography in the initial evaluation of asymptomatic microhematuria. *J Urol*; 168: 2457-2460.

[114] Warshauer DM, McCarthy SM, Street SM, et al. (1988). Detection of renal masses: sensitivities and specificities of excretory urography/linear tomography, US, and CT. *Radiology*; 169: 363.

[115] Dikranian AH, Pettiti DB, Shapiro CE, et al. (2005). Intravenous urography in evaluation of asymptomatic microhematuria. *J Endourol* (19)5: 595-597.

[116] Lang E, Macchia RJ, Thomas R, et al. (2003). Improved detection of renal pathologic features on multiphasic helical CT compared with IVU in patients presenting with microscopic hematuria. *Urology* (61)3: 528-532.

[117] Schulam PG, Kawashima A, Sandler C, et al. Urinary Tract Imaging-Basic Principles. In Walsh PC, Retik AB, Vaughan Jr. ED, Wein AJ eds. *Campbell's Urology 8th Edition*, Philadelphia: Saunders, 2002:122-166.

[118] Mucksavage P, Kutikov A, Magerfleisch L, et al. (2011). Comparison of radiological imaging modalities for measuring the diameter of renal masses: is there a sizeable difference? *BJU int; Epub.*

[119] Bos SD and Mensink HJ. (1998). Can duplex Doppler ultrasound replace computerized tomography in staging patients with renal cell carcinoma? *Scand J Urol Nephrol.*: (2):87-91.

[120] Karam JA, Ahrar K, Matin SF. (2011). Ablation of kidney tumors. *Surg Oncol Clin N Am*. 20: 341-353.

[121] Jamis-Dow CA, Choyke PL, Jennings SB, et al. (1996). Small (<or= 3 –cm) renal masses: detection with CT versus US and pathologic correlation. *Radiology*, 198: 785-788.

[122] Girard MS, Mattrey RF, Baker KG, et al. (2000). Comparison of standard and second harmonic B-mode sonography in the detection of segmental renal infarction with sonographic contrast in a rabbit model. *J Ultrasound Med;* 19: 185-192.

[123] Tamai, H, Takiguchi Y, MT, Oka M et al. (2005). Contrast-Enhanced Ultrasonography in the Diagnosis of Solid Renal Tumors. *J Ultrasound Med* (24):1635-1640.

[124] Park BK, Kim B, Kim SH, et al. (2007). Assessment of renal cystic masses based on Bosniak classification: comparison of CT and contrast-enhanced US. *Eur J Radiol.* 61;: 310-314.

[125] Quaia E, Bertolotto M, Cioffi V, et al. (2008). Comparison of contrast-enhanced sonography with unenhanced sonography and contrast-enhanced CT in the diagnosis of malignancy in complex cystic renal masses. *AJR Am J Roentgenol.* 191: 1239-1249.

[126] Ascenti G, Gaeta M, Magno C, et al. (2004). Contrast-enhanced second-harmonic sonography in the detection of pseudocapsule in renal cell carcinoma. *AJR Am J Roentgenol.* 182: 1525-1530.

[127] Correas JM, Claudon M, Tranquart F, et al. (2006). The kidney: imaging with microbubble contrast agents. *Ultrasound Q*. 22. 53-66-178.

[128] Tamai H, TakiguchiY, Oka M, et al. (2005). Contrast-enhanced ultrasonography in the diagnosis of solid renal tumors. *J Ultrasound Med;* 24: 1635-1640.

[129] Piscaglia F and Bolondi L. (2006). The safety of Sonovue in abdominal applications: retrospective analysis of 23,188 investigations. *Ultrasound Med Biol;* 32: 1369-1375.

[130] Israel GM and Bosniak MA. Renal Imaging for diagnosis and staging of renal cell carcinoma. In Taneja SS ed. *Contemporary management of renal cell carcinoma.* Philadelphia: W. B. Saunders Company, 2003: 30; 499-514.

[131] Brenner DJ and Hall EJ. (2007). Computed tomography—an increasing source of radiation exposure. *N Engl J Med.* 357, 2277-2284.

[132] Ruile P. improved computed tomography system marketed. (2008). *Medical News Today.*

[133] Schulam PG, Kawashima A, Sandler C, et al. Urinary Tract Imaging-Basic Principles. In Walsh PC, Retik AB, Vaughan Jr. ED, Wein AJ eds. *Campbell's Urology* 8th *Edition,* Philadelphia: Saunders, 2002:122-166.

[134] Sheth S and Fishman EK. CT in Kidney Cancer. *Imaging of Kidney Cancer.* New York: Springer Berlin Heidelberg 2006: 29-49.

[135] Israel GM, Bosniak MA. (2005). How I do it: evaluating renal masses. *Radiology;* 236: 441-450.

[136] Birnbaum BA, Hindman N, Lee J, et al. (2007). Renal cyst pseudoenhancement: influence of multidetector CT reconstruction algorithm and scanner type in phantom model. *Radiology;* 244: 767-775.

[137] Lockhart ME and Smith K. Technical considerations in renal CT. In Kenney PJ. ed. *Radiologic Clinics of North America- Advances in Renal Imaging.* Philadelphia, Pennsylvania, W. B. Saunders Company, 2003. 41 (5):863-875.

[138] Leschka S, Stolzmann P, Baumuller S, et al. (2010). Performance of dual-energy CT with tin filter technology for the discrimination of renal cysts and enhancing masses. *Acad Radiol;* 17: 526-534.

[139] Graser A, Becker CR, Staehler M, et al. (2010). Single-phase dual energy CT allows for characterization of renal masses as benign or malignant. *Invest Radiol*; 45: 399-405.

[140] Miles KA. (2002). Functional computed tomography in oncology. *Eur J Cancer*; 38:2079-2084.

[141] Kambadakone AR, Sahani DV. (2009). Body perfusion CT: technique, clinical applications, and advances. *Radiol Clin North AM*; 47: 161-178.

[142] Ng CS, Wang X, Faria SC, et al. (2010). Perfusion CT in patients with metastatic renal cell carcinoma treated with interferon. *AJR*; 194: 166-171.

[143] Gigli F, Zattoni F, ZamboniG, et al. (2010). Correlation between pathologic features and perfusion CT of renal cancer: a feasibility study. *Urologia*; 77: 223-231.

[144] Bosniak MA, Megibow AJ, Hulnick DH, et al. (1998). CT diagnosis of renal angiomyolipoma: The importance of detecting small amounts of fat. *AJR Am J Roentgenol*; 151:497-501.

[145] Henderson RJ, Germany R, Peavy PW, et al. (1997). Fat density in renal cell carcinoma: Demonstration with computerized tomography. *J Urol*; 157:1347-1348.

[146] Milner J, McNeil B, Proud K, et al. (2005). Fat poor renal angiomyolipoma: Patient and imaging characteristics. *J Urol*; 173:266.

[147] Milner J, McNeil B, Alioto J, et al. (2006). Fat Poor Renal Angiomyolipoma: Patient, Computerized Tomography and Histological Findings. *J Urol*; 176(3): 905-909.

[148] Kang SK, Kim D, and Chandara H. (2011). Contemporary imaging of the renal mass. *Cur Urol Rep*; 12:11-17.

[149] Davenport MS, Neville AM, Ellis JH, et al. (2011). Diagnosis of renal angiomyolipomas with Hounsfield unit thresholds: effect of size of region of interest and nephrographic phase imaging. *Radiology*; 260; 158-165.

[150] Sheir KZ, El-Azab M, Mosbah A, et al. (2005) Differentiation of renal cell carcinoma subtypes by multislicecomputerized tomography. *J Urol*; 174(2):451–455.

[151] Kim JK, Kim TK, Ahn HJ, et al. (2002) Differentiation of subtypes of renal cell carcinoma on helical CT scans. AJR *Am J Roentgenol;* 178(6):1499–1506.

[152] Dunnick NR, Sandler CM, Amis Jr ES, et al. *Textbook of Uroradiology*. Baltimore, Maryland. Williams & Wilkins, 1997: 44-85.

[153] Hecht EM, Israel GM, Krinsky GA, et al. (2004). Renal Masses: Quantitative Analysis of enhancement with signal intensity measurements versus qualitative analysis of enhancement with image subtraction for diagnosing malignancy at MR imaging. *Radiology*; 232: 373-378.

[154] Terens WL, Gluck R, Golimbu M, et al. (1992). Use of gadolinium DTPA-enhanced MRI to characterize renal mass in patient with renal insufficiency. *Urology* (40): 152-154.

[155] Nelson KL, Gifford LM, Lauber-Huber C, et al. (1995). Clinical safety of gadopentate dimeglumine. *Radiology* (196): 439-443.

[156] Prince MR, Arnoldus C, and Frisoli JK. (1996). Nephrotoxicity of high dose gadolinium compared with iodinated contrast. *J Magn Reson Imaging*; 6: 162-6.

[157] Rofsky NM, Weinreb JC, Bosniak MA, et al. (1991). Renal lesion characterization with gadolinium-enhanced MR imaging: efficacy and safety in patients with renal insufficiency. *Radiology*; 180: 85-89.

[158] Zhang J, Pedrosa I, and Rofsky NM. MR techniques for renal imaging. In Kenney PJ. ed. *Radiologic Clinics of North America- Advances in Renal Imaging*. Philadelphia, Pennsylvania, W. B. Saunders Company, 2003. 41: (5):877-907.

[159] Natalin R, Prince M, Grossman M, et al. (2010). Contemporary applications and limitations of magnetic resonance imaging contrast materials. *J Urol*; 183: 27-33.

[160] Ho VB and Choyke PL. MR evaluation of solid renal masses. In Lee VS ed. *Magnetic Resonace Imaging Clinics of North America-Genitourinary MR Imaging.* Philadelphia. W. B. Saunders. 2004; (12) 413-427.

[161] Taouli B, Thakur RK, Mannelli L, et al. (2009). Renal lesions: characterization with diffusion-weighted imaging versus contrast enhanced contrastenhanced MR imaging. *Radiology*, 251:398–407.

[162] Zhang J, Tehrani YM, Wang L, et al. (2008). Renal masses: characterization with diffusion-weighted MR Imaging: a preliminary experience. *Radiology*, 247:458–464.

[163] Rosenkrantz AB, Niver BE, Fitzgerald EF, et al. (2010). Utility of the apparent diffusion coefficient for distinguishing clear cell renal cell carcinoma of low and high nuclear grade. *AJR Am J Roentgenol.* 195: W344-351.

[164] Inci E, Hocaoglu E, Aydin S, et al. (2011). Diffusion-weighted magnetic resonance imaging in evaluation of primary solid and cystic renal masses using the Bosniak classification. Eur J Radiol. March. Epub.

[165] Gabr AH, Gdor Y, Roberts W, et al: Radiographic surveillance of minimally and moderately complex renal cysts. (2009). *BJU Int*; 103: 1116-1119.

[166] Israel GM, Hindman N, Hecht E, et al. (2005). The use of opposed-phase chemical shift MRI in the diagnosis of renal angiomyolipomas. *AJR Am J Roentgenol*; 184: 1868-1872.

[167] Choi HJ, Kim JK, Kim CS, et al. (2011). Value of t2 weighted MR imaging in differentiating low-fat renal angiomyolipomas from other renal tumors. *Acta Radiol*; 52: 349-353.

[168] Harmon WJ, King BF, Lieber MM. (1996). Renal oncocytoma: Magnetic resonance imaging characteristics. *J Urol*;155:863-867.

[169] Perkins AC and Missailidis. (2007). Radiolabelled aptamers for tumor imaging and therapy. *Q J Nucl Med Mol Imaging*; 51: 292-296.

[170] Gormley TS, Van Every MJ, Moreno AJ. (1996). Renal oncocytoma: Preoperative diagnosis using technetium 99m sestamibi imaging. *Urology*;48:33-39.

[171] Rohren EM, Turkington TG, Coleman RE. (2004). Clinical applications of PET in oncology. *Radiology.*;231:305–332.

[172] Jarritt PH, Carson KJ, Hounsell AR, et al. (2006). The role of PET/CT scanning in radiotherapy planning. *Br J Radiol.*; 79:27–35.

[173] Rigo P, Paulus P, Kaschten BJ, et al. (1996). Oncological applications of positron emission tomography with fluorine-18 fluorodeoxyglucose. *Eur J Nucl Med.*;23:1641–1674.

[174] Glaspy JA, Hawkins R, Hoh CK, et al. (1993). Use of positron emission tomography in oncology. *Oncology*;7:41–50.

[175] Flier JS, Mueckler MM, Usher P, et al. (1987). Elevated levels of glucose transport and transporter messenger RNA are induced by ras or src oncogenes. *Science*;235:1492–1495.

[176] Monakhov NK, Neistadt EL, Shavlovskil MM, et al. (1978). Physicochemical properties and isoenzyme composition of hexokinase from normal and malignant human tissues. *J Natl Cancer Inst*; 61:27–34.

[177] Kocher F, Geimmel S, Hauptmann R, et al. (1994). Preoperative lymph node staging in patients with kidney and urinary bladder neoplasm. *J Nucl* Med.; 35:223.

[178] Ramdave S, Thomas GW, Berlangieri SU, et al. (2001). Clinical role of F-18 fluorodeoxyglucose positron emission tomography for detection and management of renal cell carcinoma. *J Urol;* 166:825–830.

[179] Ozulker T, Ozulker F, Ozbek E, et al: (2011). A prospective diagnostic accuracy study of F-18 fluorodeoxyglucose-positron emission tomography/computed tomography in the evaluation of indeterminate renal masses. *Nucl Med Commun; 32: 265-272.*

[180] Aide N, Cappele O, Bottet P, et al. (2003). Efficiency of [^{18}F]FDG PET in characterising renal cancer and detecting distant metastases: a comparison with CT. *Eur J Nucl Med Mol Imaging*; 30:1236–1245.

[181] Blake MA, McKernan M, Setty B, et al. (2006). Renal oncocytoma displaying intense activity on ^{18}F-FDG PET. *Am J Roentgenol;* 186:269–270.

[182] Goldberg MA, Mayo-Smith WW, Papanicolaou N, et al. (1997). FDG PET characterization of renal masses: preliminary experience. *Clin Radiol;* 52:510–515.

[183] Baert J, Vandamme B, Sciot R, et al. (1995) Benign angiomyolipoma involving the renal vein and vena cava as a tumor thrombus: case report. *J Urol;* 153: 1205-1207.

[184] Rasalkar DD, Chu WC, Chan AW, et al: (2011) Malignant pigmented clear cell epitheloid cell tumor (PEComa) in an adolescent boy with widespread metastases: a rare entity in this age group. *Pediatr Radiol.* May 2011 Epub ahead of print.

[185] Khan MS, Iram S, O'Brien TS, et al: (2006) Renal " Perivascular Epitheloid Cell-omas". *BJU Int;* 98:1146-1147.

[186] Ponholzer A, Reiter WJ, and Maier U. (2002) Organ sparing surgery for giant bilateral renal oncocytoma. *J. Urol;* 2002: 2531-2532.

[187] Akbulut S, Senol A, Cakabay B, et al. (2010) Giant renal oncocytoma: a case report and review of the literature. *J Med Case Reports;* 17: 52-56.

[188] Jinzaki M, Mctavish JD, Zou KH, et al. (2004) Evaluation of small (</= 3 cm) renal masses with MDCT: benefits of thin overlappingreconstructions. *AJR Am J Roentgenol;* 183: 223-228.

[189] Jinzaki M and Kuribayashi S. (2007)Re: Dynamic contrast –enhanced CT of renal cell carcinoma for evaluation of tumor vascularity: analysis of single-phase or multiphase scanning. *AJR Am J Roentgeno;l* 2007; 188: 569.

[190] Campbell SC, Novick AC , and RM Bukowski: Renal tumors. In Wein AJ, Kavoussi LR, Novick AC, Partin AW, and Peters CA ed: Campbell-walsh urology 9th Ed. Philadelphia, Saunders Elseiver. 2007: 1567-1637.

2

Tubulocystic Carcinoma of the Kidney, a Rare Distinct Entity

Shreenath Bishu, Laurie J. Eisengart and Ximing J. Yang*
Department of Pathology, Northwestern University, Feinberg School of Medicine, Feinberg, Chicago, IL USA

1. Introduction

Tubulocystic carcinoma is a rare renal tumor with distinct characteristics which were recently described in details in three large series (1, 2, 3). Tubulocystic carcinomas of the kidney well circumscribed tumors. They are usually solitary and are composed of closely packed tubules and cysts separated by fibrous stroma and lined by a single layer of cuboidal cells with eosinophilic cytoplasm and prominent nucleoli, sometimes with a hobnail appearance. These tumors show a low but definite risk of metastasis, and it is therefore important to distinguish them from other benign and malignant renal lesions included in the differential diagnosis.

Tubulocystic carcinoma was originally described as a subtype of collecting duct carcinoma (4). Carcinoma of the collecting duct of Bellini, first described by Pierre Masson (5) and characterized by a tubular or tubulopapillary growth pattern with high grade nuclei, follows an aggressive clinical course with a very poor prognosis. When tubulocystic carcinoma was first described, it was included in a series of 13 cases called "low grade collecting duct carcinoma" (4); these tumors feature a favorable clinical outcome distinct from high grade collecting duct carcinoma of the kidney. The entity "low grade collecting duct carcinoma" was later divided into two distinct subtypes, mucinous tubular and spindle cell carcinoma (6-8) and tubulocystic carcinoma (5). While mucinous tubular and spindle cell carcinoma is now recognized as a distinct subtype of renal cell carcinoma (RCC) in the World Health Organization classification system of renal tumors (WHO) (3), tubulocystic carcinoma is still being characterized (1, 2, 3, 9) and is not yet included in the current WHO classification system. Mounting morphologic, biologic, immunohistochemical, and molecular evidence supports that this tumor represents a unique subtype of RCC (1, 2, 3).

2. Clinical presentation and epidemiology

In the majority of cases, the tumor is discovered incidentally. Less commonly, a patient with tubulocystic carcinoma of the kidney may present with nonspecific abdominal pain, a flank mass, distention, gross hematuria or unintentional weight loss as in reported cases (1, 4, 9).

---

* Correspondig Author

Tubulocystic carcinoma occurs in the 4th through the 9th decades of life. Patients range in age from 30 to 80 years in the 64 reported cases (1, 2, 3, 9), with an overall mean age of 57.2 years. Tubulocystic carcinoma arises in men in the vast majority of cases, with an overall male to female ratio of 7:1.

3. Gross pathology

Tubulocystic carcinomas are well circumscribed masses composed of multilocular cystic spaces, some containing serous fluid. The cut surface is characteristically described as "bubble-wrap", "spongy" or "Swiss cheese" in appearance due to the multiple cystic spaces. The tumors typically do not show areas of solid growth, and hemorrhage or necrosis is uncommon. The reported sizes of these tumors have ranged from 0.5 to 17.5cm with an overall mean of 4.3cm. The majority of the tumors involve the renal cortex or the cortex and medulla (1, 2, 3, 9), not the medulla alone, which would be the typical location of a collecting duct carcinoma.

In the majority of recently studied cases (51 of 64), tubulocystic carcinoma arises as a single nodule. Yang et al. reported 5 of 13 cases were associated with papillary renal cell neoplasms.

4. Histology

The tumors are composed of variably sized, closely packed tubules and cysts separated by thin fibrous septae. There is no ovarian-type stroma or desmoplasia in the fibrous septae. The cysts typically range from 0.05 to 2mm, but can be as large as 1 cm (1, 3). Areas of papillary architecture or solid growth are not identified unless the tumor is associated with papillary cell neoplasms. The tubules and cysts are lined by a single layer of cuboidal cells with eosinophilic cytoplasm (Figure 1). A hobnail morphology is characteristic. Nucleoli are typically prominent, and the majority of cases would be graded as Fuhrman nuclear grade 3. Although we typically do not grade tubulocystic carcinoma with Fuhrman grading system since this tumor is biologically low grade. Mitoses are rare or absent. Necrosis or lymphovascular invasion is usually not identified.

One of the common findings associated with tubulocystic carcinoma is the coexisting papillary renal cell neoplasms. In the previous study, tubulocystic carcinoma was found adjacent to and/or intermingled with papillary renal cell carcinoma (RCC) and papillary adenoma in 4 of 15 cases, and 1 was found in conjunction with papillary carcinomatosis (3). The associated papillary RCC can be type 1 or type 2 (Figure 2). The findings have been substantiated with more cases in our experience although other series have not reported tubulocystic carcinoma in association with other forms of RCC (1, 2, 4, 9).

5. Differntial diagnosis

The differential diagnosis includes simple cortical cyst, cystic nephroma, multilocular cystic RCC, and mixed epithelial and stromal tumor of the kidney.

Simple cortical cysts

Simple cortical cysts are not multilocular, and the lining cells resemble normal renal tubules.

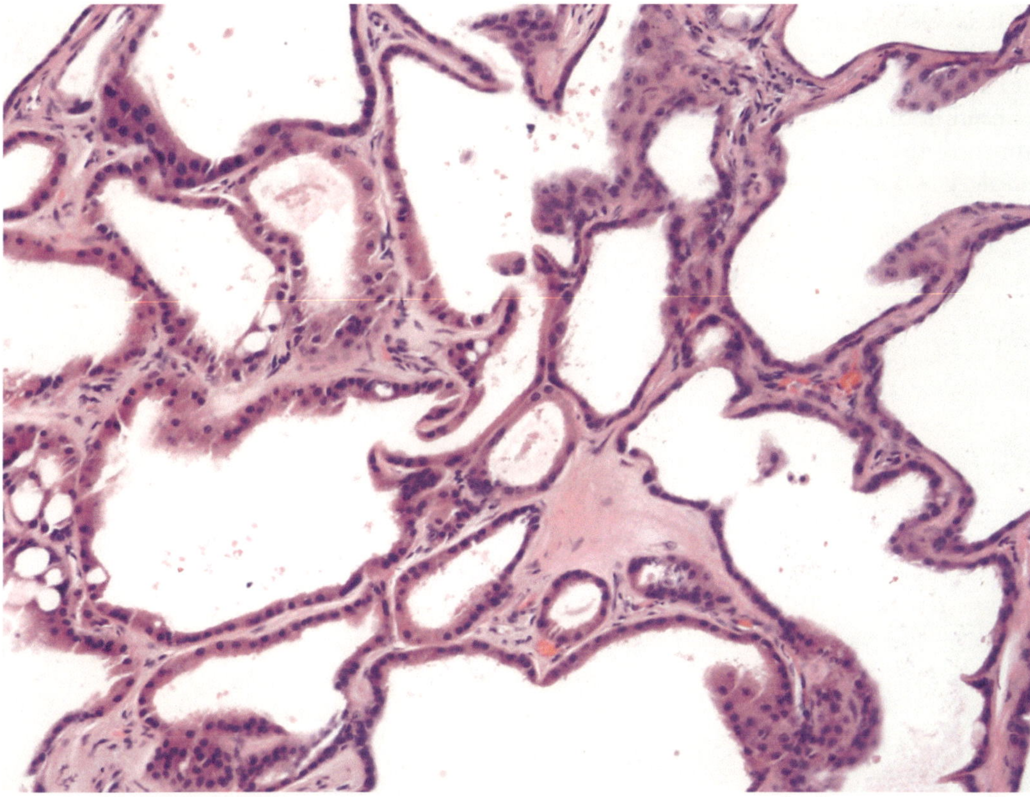

Fig. 1. Tubulocystic carcinoma is composed of cystic structures lined by tumor cells with eosinophilic cytoplasm and prominent nucleoli.

Cystic nephroma

Cystic nephroma can be multiloculated and lined by a single layer of epithelial cells. The lining epithelium is composed of flattened or attenuated cells; there may be hobnailing. However, significant nuclear atypia is absent and nucleoli are not prominent. Also cystic nephroma may have ovarian-type of stroma.

Mixed epithelial and stromal tumor

Mixed epithelial and stromal tumor of the kidney can be distinguished by the presence of stromal proliferation in the septae and variable histology of the cyst lining cells, which are typically not high nuclear grade.

Multilocular cystic renal cell carcinoma

The cysts of multilocular cystic RCC are lined by clear cells similar to clear cell RCC, without eosinophilic cytoplasm or high nuclear grade; nests of clear cells are also present in the walls of the cysts.

6. Immunohistochemistry

Tubulocystic carcinoma is positive for CD10 and AMACR (P504S), and shows weak or heterogeneous staining for CK7 (2, 10). Strong staining is seen for CK8, CK18 and CK19 (1, 2,

9). It is also positive for Pax2, kidney specific cadherin, carbonic anhydrase IX, and parvalbumin (1). There have been mixed reports of the expression of high molecular weight cytokeratin and UEA-1 (1, 2, 9, 11). This mixture of expression of proximal and distal nephron markers argues against origin from the collecting duct system. Yang et al. have proposed that the AMACR and CK7 expression, along with other features (see *Gross Pathology* and *Molecular Characteristics*) suggests a relationship with papillary RCC.

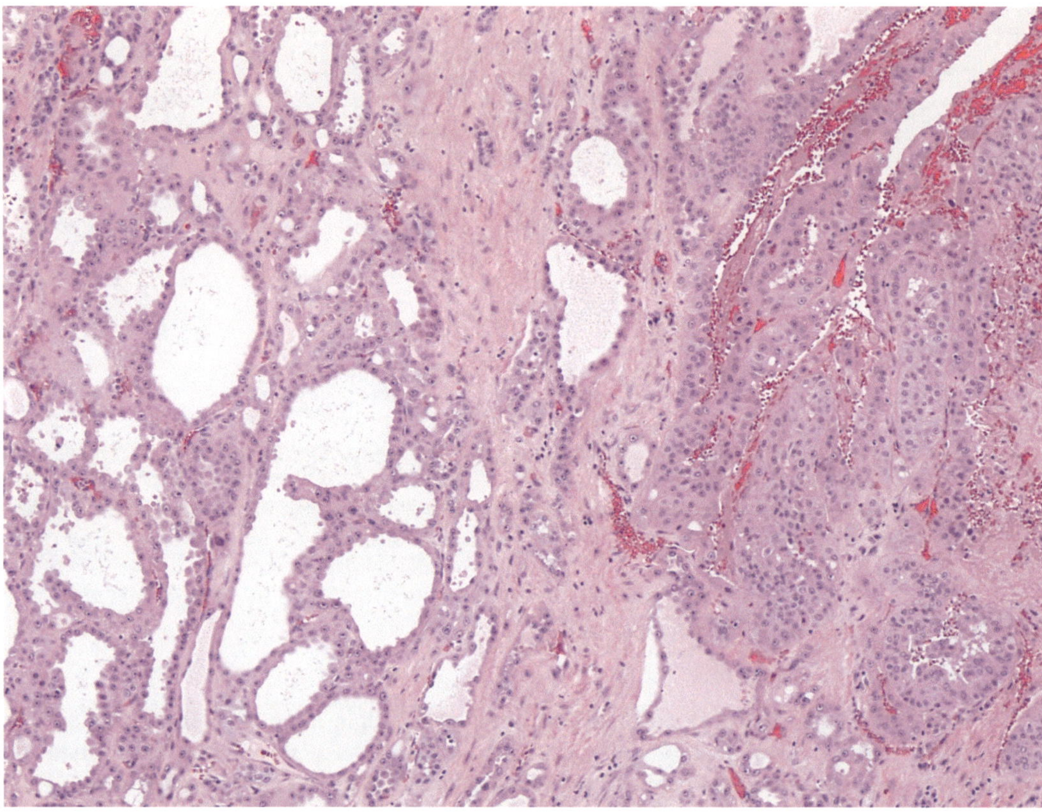

Fig. 2. Co-existing tubulocystic carcinoma (on the left side) and type 2 papillary RCC, high grade (on the right side) of the photo.

7. Ultrastructural features

Amin et al. report that electron microscopy of tubulocystic carcinoma reveals features of both proximal convoluted tubules and intercalated cells of the collecting duct (1). Abundant microvilli with brush border organization was reminiscent of proximal convoluted tubules. A few cells showed shorter, sparse microvilli with cytoplasmic interdigitation, corresponding to intercalated cells. Mitochondria are abundant in tumor cells (1, 9).

8. Molecular features

Yang et al. demonstrated a unique molecular signature of tubulocystic carcinoma in comparison to other renal tumors (n = 55) and normal renal tissue using gene expression microarray analysis. Clustering analysis of that data revealed tubulocystic carcinoma to be closely related to papillary RCC; both types 1 and 2 dimensional clustering placed tubulocystic carcinoma between low and high grade papillary RCC. Comparative genomic microarray analysis was performed and demonstrated gains of chromosome 17p and 17q (trisomy 17), similar to papillary RCC. Gains of chromosome 7p and 7q (trisomy 7), also characteristic of papillary RCC, were not identified in the one case of tubulocystic carcinoma studied (3).

A recent study by Zhou et al on tubulocystic carcinoma and papillary RCC was performed by multicolor fluorescence in situ hybridization (FISH) assay containing probes for chromosomes 7, 17, and Y. Typically papillary RCCs have frequent loss of chromosome Y, and gains of chromosomes 7 and 17 (trisomies 7 and 17). Particularly chromosome 17 gain is believed to be relatively specific for papillary RCC, as previously reported in 93% to 100% of papillary RCC (12). This study by Zhou et al showed that 10/12 (83%) cases of tubulocystic carcinoma had chromosome 7 gains, while only 8/12 (66.7%) cases had chromosome 17 gains, and 8/9 cases had the Y chromosome loss. The findings suggested a strong genetic similarity between tubulocytic carcinoma and papillary RCC. However, they are not identical in the cytogenetic changes, since one third of tubulocytic carcinomas cases did not demonstrated typical gains of chromosome 17, which are relatively specific for papillary RCC.

Using gene expression profiling, Amin et al. found differential expression of genes related to cell cycle and biomolecule metabolism when compared to clear cell and chromophobe RCC- the origin from the collecting duct of Bellini. However, the findings suggest that tubulocytic carcinoma is a distinct subtype of renal cell carcinoma, no papillary RCCs were included in the comparison (1).

Recently, Osunkoya et al.compared mRNA expression of several genes in tubulocystic and collecting duct carcinomas. The genes were chosen in light of immunohistochemical characterization of these tumors (see *Immunohistochemistry*). Tubulocystic carcinomas showed relative overexpression of vimentin, p53 and AMACR. While not statistically significant, tubulocystic carcinoma tended to have higher levels of E-cadherin and CD10, and lower levels of CK19. CK7 and parvalbumin expression were not different between the two groups 13).

9. Clinical outcome and prognosis

The majority of tumors (50/64) have been stage T1 at presentation; 9 were stage T2 and 5 were T3 (1, 2, 3, 9, 11). Where tumors were discovered antemortem, treatment was with total or partial nephrectomy (1, 2, 3, 9 11) .

Where available, clinical follow-up has ranged from 3 to104 months. The vast majority of patients did not experience recurrence or metastasis, and were alive with no evidence of disease. MacLennan et al. report one patient who died of widespread intraabdominal metastasis 46 months after diagnosis (11). Yang et al. reported one patient with pelvic lymph node metastasis at nephrectomy that the metastatic tumor was histologically identical to the primary, but no evidence of disease with limited follow-up (3). Other patients in that series did show metastatic disease from their concurrent papillary RCC. In the series by Amin et al, one patient developed local recurrence and two developed distant metastasis, one to liver and both to bone (1). All the patients in the series by Azoulay et al. had no evidence of recurrence or metastasis (2).

Overall, tubulocystic carcinomas have a small but definite risk for metastasis, and are best considered a low malignant tumor. This risk is markedly increased when tubulocystic carcinoma is associated with high grade papillary RCC.

10. Conclusion

Tubulocystic carcinoma is a rare renal tumor with distinct characteristics. Although originally described as a low grade collecting duct carcinoma, the biologic behavior, immunohistochemical profile, and molecular signature of these tumors do not support origin from the collecting ducts of Bellini, and suggests that they are a distinct subtype of renal cell carcinoma, with a close relationship to papillary renal cell carcinoma. This relationship has been observed in a subset of tubulocystic carcinoma and needs further investigation. These tumors show a low but definite risk of metastasis, and it is therefore important to distinguish them from other renal lesions in the differential diagnosis.

11. References

[1] Amin MB, MacLennan GT, Gupta R, et al. Tubulocystic carcinoma of the kidney: clinicopathologic analysis of 31 cases of a distinctive rare subtype of renal cell carcinoma. *Am J Surg Pathol.* 2009;33:384-392.

[2] Azoulay S, Vieillefond A, Paraf F, et al. Tubulocystic carcinoma of the kidney: a new entity among renal tumors. *Virchows Arch.* 2007;451:905-909.

[3] Yang XJ, Zhou M, Hes O, et al. Tubulocystic carcinoma of the kidney: clinicopathologic and molecular characterization. *Am J Surg Pathol.* 2008;32:177-187.

[4] MacLennan GT, Farrow GM, Bostwick DG. Low-grade collecting duct carcinoma of the kidney: report of 13 cases of low-grade mucinous tubulocystic renal carcinoma of possible collecting duct origin. *Urology.* 1997;50:679-684.

[5] Masson P. *Tumeurs Humaines 1955. Human Tumors, Histology, Diagnosis and Technique.* Detroit: Wayne State University Press; 1970.

[6] Parwani AV, Husain AN, Epstein JI, et al. Low-grade myxoid renal epithelial neoplasms with distal nephron differentiation. *Hum Pathol.* 2001;32:506-512.

[7] Srigley JR, Eble JN, Grignon DJ. Unusual renal cell carcinoma (RCC) with prominent spindle cell change possibly related to the loop of Henle. *Modern Pathology.* 1999;12:107A.

[8] Srigley JR, Kapusta L, Reuter V. Phenotypic, molecular, and ultrastructural studies of a novel low grade renal epithelial neoplasm possibly related to the loop of Henle. *Modern Pathology.* 2002;15:182A.

[9] Farah R, Ben-Izhak O, Munichor M, et al. Low-grade renal collecting duct carcinoma. A case report with histochemical, immunohistochemical, and ultrastructural study. *Ann Diagn Pathol.* 2005;9:46-48.

[10] Eble JN SG, Epstein JI. *Pathology and Genetics of Tumors of the Urinary System and Male Genital Organs.* Lyon: IARC Press; 2004.

[11] MacLennan GT, Bostwick DG. Tubulocystic carcinoma, mucinous tubular and spindle cell carcinoma, and other recently described rare renal tumors. *Clin Lab Med.* 2005;25:393-416.

[12] Zhou M, Yang XJ, Lopez J. Renal tubulocystic carcinoma is closely related to papillary renal cell carcinoma: implications for pathologic classification. *Am J Surg Pathol.* 2009.

[13] Osunkoya AO, Young AN, Wang W, et al. Comparison of Gene Expression Profiles in Tubulocystic Carcinoma and Collecting Duct Carcinoma of the Kidney. *Am J Surg Pathol.* 2009.

3

Active Surveillance of Renal Cortical Neoplasms

Adam C. Mues[1], Joseph A. Graversen[2] and Jaime Landman[2]
[1]*New York University School of Medicine, Department of Urology,*
[2]*University of California Irvine Medical Center, Department of Urology,*
USA

1. Introduction

Over the last two decades there has been an increase in the detection of small (≤ 4 cm) renal cortical neoplasms (RCN) that is attributed to the increase in axial abdominal imaging.[1] Although these lesions are typically asymptomatic in nature, they present a potential management dilemma for the treating urologist. The standard of management in kidney cancer has always been surgical excision with either radical nephrectomy or partial nephrectomy. For tumors <4.0cm, partial nephrectomy is now the surgical standard, which provides equivalent cancer control compared with radical nephrectomy and provides a nephron-sparing treatment.[2]

Historically, the majority of incidental renal masses have been treated relatively soon after detection. While effective, this treatment paradigm has limited our knowledge regarding the natural history of the small renal mass. It has also been observed that despite the increase in the detection of renal cell carcinoma (RCC), that there has not been a significant impact on patient overall survival.[3] Therefore, it is necessary to explore the concept of active surveillance (AS) in small renal masses in order to report the observed natural history and use this knowledge to make accurate and appropriate treatment recommendations to patients. Previously, AS was recommended only for patients with a reduced life expectancy such as the elderly or in patients at high risk for a surgical procedure. Currently, AS is also utilized for healthy patients who reject surgical management or a renal ablation procedure.[2] This chapter will review the natural history of the small renal mass, factors to consider when recommending active surveillance, contemporary treatment outcomes, and the role of the image-guided renal mass biopsy.

2. Natural history

The natural history refers to the behavior of the small renal mass over time with no intervention. The critical questions to be addressed are: can tumors metastasize? When do they metastasize? How do patients know if their tumor is the type that will metastasize? Table 1 shows data from 11 of the larger AS series, which provides some insight into the natural history of these tumors. However the most series are retrospective and vary in terms of selection criteria for inclusion and renal mass monitoring, which introduces selection bias. Therefore, the lack of prospective randomized controlled trials limit the interpretation of the data regarding AS to some degree. Rendon and colleagues followed 13 tumors with a mean follow-up of 30.7 months and observed a mean GR of 0.22cm/year. There was no progression to metastatic disease.[4] Volpe and coworkers followed 32 tumors in 29 patients for a mean time of 39 months. The mean tumor size was 2.5cm with a mean growth rate of 0.1cm/year. There were no deaths or cases progressing to metastasis.[5] However, most of the literature is composed of small retrospective single center studies with small patient cohorts and short-term follow-up. The majority of tumors on AS are small (≤ 4cm) providing no knowledge about the natural history of larger tumors. In addition, there is no standard in terms of inclusion criteria, surveillance protocol or time for delayed intervention. A meta-analysis in 2006 from 9 different centers observed 234 tumors with a mean size of 2.6cm and an average growth rate of 0.28cm/year. There were 56% of tumors with available pathology and 92% were found to be renal cell carcinoma (RCC). These confirmed RCC lesions grew at a rate of 0.4cm/year, which is considerably faster than the lesions remaining on AS (0.2cm/yr).[6] Recently, the largest single center study on AS demonstrated an average GR of 0.34cm/yr in 223 tumors followed for 35 months. Eleven (5%) patients required some form of delayed intervention. There were 4 patients that progressed to metastatic disease and 1 cancer-specific death.[7]

3. Review of management options for the cT1 renal mass

Historically, the gold standard for the treatment of renal masses of any size was radical nephrectomy. However, the importance of nephron-sparing surgery focuses not only on avoiding chronic renal insufficiency, but also to decrease the incidence of cardiovascular events and death.[8,9,10] Therefore, in patients with a renal mass ≤ 4cm (cT1a), partial nephrectomy is the new gold standard. It has even been suggested that tumors <7cm (cT1b) should be managed with parital nephrectomy when surgically feasible.[2] In addition, the use of minimally invasive techniques should be applied when possible to improve patient related benefits such as reduced post-operative pain, shorter hospital stay and a faster post-operative recovery. In addition to partial nephrectomy, renal tumors can be ablated in the form of cryoablation, radiofrequency ablation (RFA), and high intensity focused ultrasound (HIFU). These modalities provide a minimally invasive treatment option for patients while avoiding surgical resection of the tumor. Both cryoablation and RFA can be performed from a laparoscopic or a percutaneous approach. The surgical approach is usually determined by tumor location with lateral and posterior tumors being treated with percutaneous ablation and anterior tumors treated with laparoscopic ablation. Percutaneous procedures do not require general anesthesia, have minimal post-operative pain, and are usually associated with a short (< 24 hour) hospital stay. Although long-term data are not yet available with these modalities, intermediate-term data demonstrates favorable recurrence and progression free survival.[11,12,13, 14]

The role of AS in the treatment of small RCN is well known and is considered a recommendation for elderly patient and in patients that are considered to be at high surgical risk. AS can be considered an option for healthy patients who have been informed of all treatment options and who insist on avoiding surgical extirpation or ablation. The majority of the urologic literature has demonstrated that most small RCNs have a slow growth rate (GR) and low risk of metastasis.[10] A summary of the contemporary AS series (820 tumors) show a growth rate of 0.27cm/year with 21% undergoing delayed intervention (Table 1). Only 12 (1.6%) lesions progressed to metastatic disease with only 1 cancer specific death. The American Urologic Association guidelines panel for the management of a T1 renal mass found that only 4 of 390 (1%) patients progressed to metastasis while on AS. This has led them to conclude that the rate of progression is sufficiently low to warrant AS in selected patients.

Active Surveillance Series	Number of patients and tumors	Mean growth rate (cm/year)	Mean follow-up (months)	Number with delayed surgery (%)	Number progressing to metastasis (%)	Cancer specific deaths (%)
Bosniak et al (1995)	37/40	0.36	39	26 (65)	0	0
Kassouf et al (2004)	24/26	0.09	32	4 (17)	0	0
Volpe et al (2004)	29/32	0.1	27.9	8 (27)	0	0
Wehle et al (2004)	29/29	0.12	32	6 (21)	0	0
Lamb et al (2004)	36/36	0.39	24	0	1 (2.8)	0
Chawla et al (2006)	49/61	0.2	36	20	1 (2)	n/a
Kouba et al (2007)	43/46	0.7	35.8	13 (30)	0	0
Abou Youssif et al (2007)	35/44	0.21	47.6	8 (23)	2 (5.7)	0
Abouassaly et al (2008)	110/110	0.26	24	4 (4)	2 (1.8)	0
Crispen et al (2009)	154/173	0.28	31	68 (44)	2 (1.8)	0
Rosales et al (2010)	212/223	0.34	35	11 (5.1)	4 (1.9)	1 (0.5)
Summary totals	**758/820**	**0.27**	**33.1**	**157 (20.7)**	**12 (1.6)**	**1**

Table 1. Summary of Active Surveillance Series

4. Active surveillance: How to decide

Initiating an AS protocol depends on the individual patient's clinical presentation. Many factors such as initial tumor size (ITS), growth rate, patient age, general medical health, and desire for intervention are considered. In addition, about 20% of small renal masses are benign and 50% to 60% are low-grade RCC.[18-20] Therefore only 20% to 30% of small RCNs are considered high-grade with aggressive features.[15-17] Frank and colleagues retrospectively reviewed 2,935 tumors from a single institution to determine if ITS was a predictive factor for malignancy. The average tumor size was 4.2cm and 6.3cm for benign and malignant tumors respectively. For each centimeter increase in diameter of the tumor, there was a 17% increase in the likelihood of the mass being malignant.[17] Additionally, larger malignant lesions were more likely to be high-grade (conventional) renal cell carcinomas (RCC) as opposed to low-grade cancers. However, the large single institution series by Rosales and colleagues and the meta-analysis by Chawla determined that there was no correlation between GR and ITS. Several series on AS have supported these findings and in general, the consensus is that ITS is not a predictive factor for an increase in GR or malignant potential in renal masses <4cm.[14,18-21]

Tumor growth rates in large single institution series and meta-analyses have been shown to be reasonably low (0.28-0.34cm/year) for most tumors.[6,7] Kunkle and co-workers concluded that there was no difference in the incidence of malignancy between tumors with zero growth versus those that do grow. However, this conclusion was based on only 6 tumors excised with no net growth over a 12 month period.[22] It is the author's firm belief that tumors with high growth rates usually represent malignant lesions and require some form of delayed intervention (DI). Crispen and colleagues found that 39% (68/173) of patients on AS underwent DI and the GR was significantly higher than those tumors that remained on AS ($p=0.023$).[23] Similarly, studies have demonstrated that GRs are significantly higher in confirmed RCC lesions compared with lesions not undergoing treatment (0.4cm/hr vs. 0.21cm/yr and 1.75cm/yr vs. 0.34cm/yr).[6,7]

Another potential predictive factor to consider when deciding on the value of an AS protocol is patient age. Abouassaly and coworkers followed an elderly population of patients (mean age 81 years) for an average of 24 months. The patients had a mean tumor size of 2.5cm and a GR of 0.26cm/yr, which are consistent finding with other contemporary series. At the conclusion of the study 31% of the cohort was deceased, however the disease specific survival was 100%.[24] A meta-analysis by Kouba and colleagues observed that there were slower tumor GRs in patients of advanced age (<60yr. had GR of 0.90 cm/yr vs. ≥60yr. had GR of 0.60 cm/yr, $p=0.057$). They also demonstrated that patients who underwent DI were significantly younger compared with those that remained on AS ($p=0.0006$). This suggests that the decision to intervene in younger patients was influenced by both GR and age.[25]

General medical fitness is another important factor when deciding on management. Patients who are high-risk for surgical related and post-operative complications or who are elderly will be better served with an active surveillance protocol or a form of ablative therapy. Many young, healthy patients prefer to be managed with a less invasive treatment as well, and elect to undergo cryoablation or radiofrequency ablation or be placed on active surveillance. Although these are not recommended as a standards or recommendations for these patients, they are options as long as the patients have been informed about risks of disease progression and the necessity of regular and careful follow-up

5. Active surveillance in large (cT1b and cT2) renal cortical neoplasms

Most urologists only consider an AS protocol for patients presenting with a cT1a (≤4cm) mass. However, there are select patients that have larger masses who may be ideal candidates for AS based on their clinical status. Mues and colleagues followed 42 tumors in 36 patients for a mean of 36 months. Average tumor size was 7.13cm and GR was 0.57cm/yr. Three patients underwent delayed intervention for rapid tumor growth. Only 2 (5.6%) patients developed metastasis and there were no cancer related deaths.[26] This data suggests that even larger masses have relatively slow growth rates with low metastatic potential.

6. Outcomes after long-term follow-up

The majority of retrospective studies have relatively short-term follow-up making it impossible to make definitive conclusions about the natural history of these tumors. Table 1 lists several AS series indicating the small number of tumors that have undergone delayed intervention, progression, or death. Abou Youssiff followed 44 tumors with a mean follow-up of 47.6 months. The average growth rate was 0.21cm/year. Two (5.7%) patients developed metastatic disease and there was 1 (2.9%) cancer specific death.[21] Haramis and colleagues reported the only single center experience with a minimum of 5 years follow-up. Fifty-one tumors with a mean follow-up of 77.1 months demonstrated a GR of 0.15cm/yr. Two (4.5%) patients had delayed intervention and there were no patients that developed metastasis or death from their tumor.[27] This represents a selected cohort due to the fact that patients with faster GR underwent DI earlier. However, the evidence suggests that tumors that are amenable to AS for a 5 year period are likely indolent and will not progress to metastatic disease or require intervention.

Patients who develop metastatic RCC generally have a poor prognosis. Large studies shows 12 reported cases on AS progressing to metastatic disease, which represents 1.6% of patients. The mean time to metastasis was 72.5 months with a mean growth rate of 1.04 cm/yr. Dechet and colleagues showed a direct correlation between tumor size and the presence of a synchronous metastasis. The authors compared 110 cases of biopsy proven metastatic RCC to 250 clinically localized tumors. As tumor size increased, there was a statistically significant increase in synchronous metastasis. They found that for every 1 cm of tumor size, the odds of finding a synchronous metastasis increased by 22%.[28] Conversely it has been shown that small tumors can also be dangerous. Minardi and co-workers followed 48 patients who had tumors after partial nephrectomy for a mean follow-up time of 92.9 months. All tumors were pT1a with clear cell renal cell carcinoma histology. Four (8.3%) developed metastatic disease at 24 months.[29] The majority of series that report metastatic disease indicate that there was interval growth in the primary lesion and that most tumors displayed an accelerated growth rate.[7,14,21,23,30,31,32] Therefore, an increased growth rate may be associated with progression to metastatic disease.

7. Role of biopsy

Until recently, renal mass biopsy has been considered unnecessary and contraindicated for the in the work-up of an enhancing solid renal mass. The procedure itself exposes the patient to potential morbidity with complications such as bleeding and hematoma formation, injury to adjacent organs, infection and pain. The false negative rate for the diagnosis of cancer is high and a sample of benign renal tissue may very well coexist with a cancerous tumor.[33] Also, there is concern related to needle biopsy tract cancer seeding with the technique itself, however there is little data to support this theory.[34] A recent study has indicated that improvements in technique have led to higher levels of diagnostic accuracy (sensitivity of 97.7% and specificity of 100%), however this practice is not considered the standard of care.[35] Rosales and co-workers performed biopsy in only 40 (19%) of their AS series.[7] However, we believe that future patients entering an AS protocol will undergo renal mass biopsy in order to optimize patient selection. New techniques such as immunohistochemical biomarkers and molecular or genomic characterization of tissue may help to identify potentially aggressive tumors that would be more likely to fail AS.

8. Conclusions

Active surveillance is a reasonable treatment option for select patients with a cT1 renal mass. Surveillance is recommended in elderly patients who either have a short life span or who are at high risk for undergoing standard surgical procedures for renal mass treatment. Active surveillance is also an option for healthy patients who do not wish to have surgery performed and who understand the risk of potential disease progression. Growth rate is likely a predictor of malignancy that should be monitored and used to determine if delayed intervention is indicated. Larger tumors (cT1b and cT2) may also be followed under AS in select patients with special attention to changes in GR. The technique and value of renal mass biopsy has changed in the last decade and now provides improved accuracy in diagnosis, which will help determine patient selection for AS protocols. Finally, long-term follow-up has improved our knowledge of the natural history of these tumors and helps urologists to better council patients in the management of their tumors.

9. References

[1] Lane BR, Novick AC. (2007). Nephron-sparing surgery. *BJU Int.* 99:1245.

[2] Novick AC, Campbell SC, Belldegrun A, et al. (2009). Guideline for management of the clinical stage 1 renal mass. American Urological Association. http://www.auanet.org/content/guidelines-and-quality-care/clinical-guidelines.cfm.

[3] Kunkle DA, Egleston BL, Uzzo RG. Excise, ablate or observe: the small renal mass dilemma--a meta-analysis and review. 2008. *J Urol* 179:1227.

[4] Rendon RA, Stanietzky N, Panzarella T, et al. (2010). The natural history of small renal masses. *J Urol* 164:1143-1147.

[5] Volpe A, Panzarella T, Rendon R, et al. (2004). The natural history of incidentally detected small renal masses. *Cancer* 738-745.

[6] Chawla AN, Crispen PL, Hanlon AL, et al. (2006). The natural history of observed enhancing renal masses: meta-analysis and review of the world literature. *J Urol* 175:425-431.

[7] Rosales JC, Haramis G, Moreno J, et al. Active surveillance of renal cortical neoplasms. *J Urol* 2010; 183:1698-1702.

[8] Huang HC, Levey, AS, Serio AM, et al. (2006). Chronic kidney disease after nephrectomy in patients with renal cortical tumors: a retrospective cohort study. *Lancet Oncol* 7:735-740.

[9] McKiernan J. Simmons R, Katz J, et al. (2006). Natural history of chronic renal insufficiency after partial and radical nephrectomy. *Urology* 59:819-820.

[10] Thompson RH, Boorjian SA, Lohse CM, et al. Radical Nephrectomy for pT1a renal masses may be associated with decreased overall survival compared with partial nephrectomy. (2008). *J Urol* 179:468-473.

[11] Desai MM, Aron M, Gill IS. (2005). Laparoscopic partial nephrectomy versus laparascopic cryoablation for the small renal tumor. *Urology* 66:23-28.

[12] Aron M, Kamoi K, Remer E, et al. (2010). Laparoscopic renal cryoablation: 8-year, single surgeon outcomes *J Urol* 183:889-895.

[13] Matin SF, Ahrar K, Cadeddu JA, et al. (2006). Residual and recurrent disease following renal energy ablative therapy: a multi-institutional study. *J Urol* 176:1973-1977.

[14] Levinson AW, Su L, Agarwal D, et al.: Long-term oncological and overall outcomes of percutaneous radio frequency ablation in high-risk surgical patients with a solitary small renal mass. *J Urol* 2008, 180: 499-504.

[15] Remzi M, Özsoy M, Klingler HC, et al. (2006). Are small renal tumors harmless? Analysis of histopathological features according to tumors 4 cm or less in diameter. *J Urol* 176:896-899.

[16] Lane BR, Babineau D, Kattan MW, et al. (2007). A preoperative nomogram for solid enhancing renal tumors 7 cm or less amenable to partial nephrectomy. *J Urol* 178:429-434.

[27] Frank I, Blute ML, Cheville JC, et al. (2003). Solid renal tumors: an analysis of pathological features related to tumor size. *J Urol* 170:2217-2220.

[18] Bosniak MA, Birnbaum BA, Krinsky GA, et al. (1995). Small renal parenchymal neoplasms: further observations on growth. *Radiology* 197:589-597.

[19] Wehle, MJ, Thiel DD, Petrou SP, et al. (2004). Conservative management of incidental contrast-enhancing renal masses as safe alternative to invasive therapy. *Urology* 64:49-52.

[20] Kouba, E, Smith A, McRacken D, et al. (2007). Watchful waiting for solid renal masses: insight into the natural history and results of delayed intervention. *J Urol* 177:466-470.

[21] Abou Youssif T, Kassouf W, Steinberg J, et al. (2007). Active surveillance for selected patients with renal masses: updated results with long-term follow-up. *Cancer* 110:1010-1014.

[22] Kunkle DA, Crispen PL, Chen DY, et al. (2007). Enhancing renal masses with zero net growth during active surveillance. *J Urol* 177:849-854.

[23] Crispin PL, Viterbo R, Boorjian SA, et al. (2009). Natural history, growth kinetics, and outcomes of untreated clinically localized renal tumors under active surveillance. *Cancer*115:2844-2852.

[24] Abouassaly R, Lane BR, Novick AC. (2008). Active surveillance of renal masses in elderly patients. *J Urol* 180:505-509.

[25] Kouba, E, Smith A, McRacken D, et al. (2007). Watchful waiting for solid renal masses: insight into the natural history and results of delayed intervention. *J Urol* 177:466-470.

[26] Mues AC, Haramis G, Badani K, et al. (2010). Active Surveillance for larger (cT1bN0M0 and cT2N0M0) renal cortical neoplasms. *Urology* 76:620-623.
[27] Haramis G, Mues AC, Rosales JC, Okhunov Z, Lanzac AP, Badani KK, Gupta M, Benson MC, McKiernan JM, Landman J. (2011). Natural history of renal cortical neoplasms during active surveillance with follow-up longer than 5 years. *Urology* 77(4):787-791.
[28] Dechet CB, Zincke H, Sebo TJ, et al. Prospective analysis of computerized tomography and needle biopsy with permanent sectioning to determine the nature of solid renal masses in adults. *J Urol* 2003;169:71-74.
[29] Minardi D, Lucarini G, Mazzucchelli R, et al. Prognostic role of Fuhrman grade and vascular endothelial growth factor in pT1a clear cell carcinoma in partial neprhectomy specimens. *J Urol* 2005; 174:1208-1212.
[30] Sowery RD, Siemens DR. Growth characteristics of renal cortical tumors in patients managed by watchful waiting. *Can J Urol* 2004;11:2407-2410.
[31] Lamb GW, Bromwich EJ, Vasey P, et al. Management of renal masses in patients medically unsuitable for nephrectomy - natural history, complications, and outcome. *Urology* 2004;64:909-913.
[32] Siu W, Hafez KS, Johnston WK, et al. Growth rates of renal cell carcinoma and oncocytoma under surveillance are similar. *Urol Oncol* 2007;25:115-119.
[33] Gill IS, Aron M, Gervais DA, et al. (2010). Small Renal Mass. *N Engl J Med* 362:624-634.
[34] Kiser GC, Totonchy M, Barry JM. (1986). Needle tract seeding after percutaneous renal adenocarcinoma aspiration. *J Urol* 136(6):1292-1293.
[35] Maturen KE, Nghiem HV, Caoili EM, et al. (2007). Renal mass core biopsy: accuracy and impact on clinical management. *AJR Am J Roentgenol* 188:563.

4

Partial Nephrectomy for the Treatment of Renal Masses: Oncologically Sound and Functionally Prudent

Eric A. Singer[1], Gopal N. Gupta[2] and Gennady Bratslavsky[1,3]
[1]*Urologic Oncology Branch, Center for Cancer Research, National Cancer Institute, National Institutes of Health, Bethesda, MD,*
[2]*Department of Urology, Loyola University Medical Center, Maywood, IL,*
[3]*Department of Urology, SUNY Upstate Medical University, Syracuse, NY, USA*

1. Introduction

The global impact of renal cell carcinoma (RCC) cannot be overemphasized. Approximately 111,100 new cases and 43,000 deaths from the disease among men in developed countries occurred in 2008 alone (Jemal et al. 2011). In 2010, RCC ranked as the seventh and eighth most common malignancy in men and women in the United States, respectively, with 58,240 new cases and 13,040 deaths expected (Jemal et al. 2010). The incidence of renal cancer has been steadily increasing over the last two decades (Chow et al. 1999; Hock et al. 2002).

Surgical extirpation is considered the gold standard for the treatment of an enhancing renal mass. This has traditionally been performed via radical nephrectomy (RN), in which the entire kidney is removed along with the renal mass. While it is possible to maintain normal renal function after a radical nephrectomy, a growing body of evidence demonstrates that there is an increasing incidence of morbidity and mortality associated with decreasing renal function. This realization has refocused attention on the importance of partial nephrectomy in the management of renal masses.

Although most of the world literature reports on the utilization of and the outcomes of sporadic RCCs, the familial renal cancer patients managed at the National Cancer Institute (NCI) provide a robust data set allowing for examination of the oncologic and renal functional outcomes of numerous clinical scenarios and technical approaches, such as initial, repeat, and salvage partial nephrectomies, as well as renal interventions performed via open, laparoscopic, or robotic approaches. While performing serial interventions on the same renal unit results in greater morbidity with each subsequent surgery, metastasis-free survival and renal replacement therapy-free survival are high, making re-operative renal surgery a reasonable option for selected patients. We now advocate that the amount of preservable renal parenchyma, rather than tumor size, be the main determinant of the feasibility of partial nephrectomy (Lane, Fergany, Linehan and Bratslavsky, 2010).

In addition to discussing the importance of surgical preservation of renal function via partial nephrectomy and its role in avoiding the morbidity and costs of renal replacement therapy (RRT), data will also be provided about emerging approaches to nephron-sparing surgery

(NSS). While open partial nephrectomy (OPN), in which only the renal mass is removed sparing the unaffected renal parenchyma, had been the only viable treatment option, advances in laparoscopic and robotic surgery have allowed for a minimally invasive approach to renal surgery that speeds convalescence and decreases the pain associated with the procedure.

In summary, this chapter will provide the rationale and oncologic and functional outcomes that support an aggressive approach towards maximal renal preservation.

2. Oncologic outcomes

2.1 Open partial nephrectomy

Current treatment guidelines issued by both the American Urological Association (AUA) and the European Association of Urology (EAU) recognize NSS as the preferred treatment for renal masses up to 7cm in size (Campbell et al. 2009; Ljungberg et al. 2010). While minimally invasive options such as laparoscopic partial nephrectomy (LPN) and robotic assisted partial nephrectomy (RAPN) are gaining in popularity, OPN provides unique advantages that have not yet been replicated by other approaches, such as the ability to use cold ischemia and non-hilar clamping to maintain a bloodless operative field (Margreiter and Marberger 2010; Volpe et al. 2011). There is robust data describing the oncologic efficacy of open partial nephrectomy (Becker et al. 2006; Becker et al. 2006; Fergany et al. 2006; Pahernik et al. 2006). (Table 1)

Author (Year)	No. of patients	Mean tumor size (cm)	5-yr CSS (%)	10-yr CSS (%)	Local recurrence (%)	Mean Follow-up (mo)
Pahernik et al (2006)	715	3	98.5	96.7	3.3	79
Becker et al (2006)	241	3.7	97.8	95.8	1.4	66
Fergany et al (2006)	400	4.2	82	-	4	62
Becker et al (2006)	69	5.3	100	100	5.8	74

Table 1. Oncologic Outcomes of Contemporary OPN Series

OPN for renal masses less than 4cm in size has been shown to be oncologically equivalent to radical nephrectomy. Belldegrun and colleagues compared 146 subjects who underwent OPN to 125 matched subjects treated with total nephrectomy and found that there was no difference in cancer-specific survival at nearly five years of follow-up (Belldegrun et al. 2008). Similarly, when comparing the cancer-specific mortality for OPN vs. radical nephrectomy in 1454 subjects treated for tumors up to 4cm at seven international academic centers, there was no statistically significant difference between the two approaches at an average follow-up of slightly more than five years (2.2% for OPN vs. 2.6% for radical nephrectomy; $p = 0.8$) (Patard et al. 2004).

Most recently, the results of the prospective, randomized EORTC phase III trial comparing the oncologic outcomes of elective NSS vs. radical nephrectomy for renal tumors up to 5cm were reported (Van Poppel et al. 2011). From 1992-2003, 541 subjects with normal contralateral renal units were enrolled and followed for a median of 9.3 years after surgery (RN = 273, NSS = 268). While this trial was closed early because of poor accrual, the overall survival rates of 81.1% for RN and 75.7% for NSS were observed. This difference was not statistically significant when analysis was limited to clinically and pathologically eligible subjects (P=0.175). Similarly, there was no significant difference in time to progression between RN and NSS (P=0.48). Cancer-specific survival was not a study endpoint and only 12 of 117 subject deaths were attributable to RCC (4 in the RN group and 8 in the NSS group).

Urologic oncologists continued to expand the "classic" non-essential indications for OPN to routinely include tumors up to 7cm in size (Russo et al. 2002; Russo 2007; Lane et al. 2010). Leibovich and colleagues retrospectively compared 91 subjects who underwent PN for tumors ranging from 4-7cm to 841 subjects treated with radical nephrectomy at the Mayo Clinic from 1970-2000 (Leibovich et al. 2004). At 5 years of follow-up, there were no statistically significant differences in cancer-specific survival and metastasis-free survival between these two groups. Dash and colleagues from Memorial Sloan-Kettering Cancer Center compared elective OPN compared elective OPN (n=45) to radical nephrectomy (n=151) in subjects with clear cell RCC tumors ranging between 4-7cm (Dash et al. 2006). They reported identical disease-free survival at 21 months of follow-up, however, the 5% recurrence rate seen in the OPN cohort prompted the authors to recommend that patients with T1b lesions managed with NSS be surveilled for an extended period of time.

2.1.1 Open partial nephrectomy for local recurrence

Obtaining a negative surgical margin is a critical objective in NSS. The size of the negative margin needed to maintain oncologic efficacy is small and the attainment of wide margins comes directly at the cost of preserved renal parenchyma (Sutherland et al. 2002). Enucleative surgery for well encapsulated tumors, in which no margin of normal parenchyma is excised, may also be a reasonable approach, especially in patients with significant pre-operative renal insufficiency or multifocal disease. This surgical approach does not appear to hamper survival outcomes compared to PNs in which a margin is taken (Carini et al. 2006; Carini et al. 2006; Minervini et al. 2011).

While surgical site recurrence rates are low and typically associated with grossly positive surgical margins at the time of NSS, the management of locally recurrent disease, or metachronous multifocal disease in the ipsilateral renal unit, is challenging and often well suited to OPN (Russo 2007). The NCI experience of managing familial renal cancer syndromes such as von Hippel-Lindau (VHL), hereditary papillary renal carcinoma (HPRC), and Birt-Hogg-Dube' (BHD) provides unique insight into the management of locally recurrent RCC (Singer and Bratslavsky 2010).

In order to preserve renal function, maximize the time interval between repeat partial nephrectomies, and minimize the risk of metastasis, the NCI employs the "3cm rule" as a size threshold for surgical decision making. When the largest solid tumor in a given kidney measures 3cm in diameter NSS is recommended via enucleation of all detectable lesions within that renal unit (Walther et al. 1999; Duffey et al. 2004). It should be noted, however, that the 3cm rule was initially developed in patients with VHL and then applied to patients with HPRC and BHD. Patients with hereditary leiomyomatosis and renal cell carcinoma (HLRCC), which is associated with papillary type 2 tumors that are known for their virulence and early metastatic potential, are never observed if solid renal tumor is detected. These patients are offered surgical extirpation that includes a margin of normal parenchyma as soon as a solid solid lesion is detected.

Re-operative NSS requires a careful balance between oncologic efficacy and renal preservation. Although there have been significant advances in the use of systemic targeted therapies to treat locally advanced and metastatic RCC, these agents are not considered curative and are associated with significant toxicities, which highlights the importance of timely and effective surgical management for local recurrences (Rini 2009).

Due to the added surgical challenges and morbidity that re-operative renal surgery entails, there are few publications available to guide patients and their oncologists (Novick and Streem 1992; Steinbach et al. 1995; Ansari et al. 2003). Johnson and colleagues at the NCI reviewed 51 planned repeat partial nephrectomies in 47 subjects with locally recurrent disease (Johnson et al. 2008). A total of 40 perioperative complications occurred. Although the majority of these complications did not result in long-term disability, one subject suffered an intraoperative myocardial infarction and died postoperatively, and three subjects lost a renal unit. Despite the increased degree of perioperative morbidity associated with repeat NSS, only 3 subjects (5.8%) in Johnson's series required RRT; a number that would have been considerably higher if radical nephrectomy had been performed, considering that one-third of the surgeries in their cohort were performed on a solitary kidney.

Bratslavsky and colleagues studied a small cohort of subjects who underwent three or more surgical interventions on the same renal unit, which they described as "salvage" PN (Bratslavsky et al. 2008). Not surprisingly, major perioperative complications occurred in 46%. However, more than 75% of the renal units were saved with minimal changes in postoperative serum creatinine, creatinine clearance, and differential renal function. The authors demonstrated that salvage PN was a viable option for select patients with recurrent, mulitifocal localized kidney cancer, and for the first time demonstrated the feasibility of such procedures, as well as resilience of the kidneys in their ability to survive repeat surgical interventions. (Table 2)

Most recently, Singer and colleagues described the renal functional and oncologic outcomes of patients with bilateral renal masses managed surgically at the NCI who had at least 10 years of post-operative follow-up (Singer et al. 2011). They identified a cohort of 128 subjects who had undergone bilateral renal surgery with a median of 3 operations per person. Sixty-eight percent of the cohort had repeat surgery on the same renal unit, with a median time between interventions of 6.2 years. At a median follow-up of 16 years, overall survival was 88%, RCC-specific survival was 97%, and metastasis-free survival was 88%. Despite bilateral, and infrequently repeat interventions, the most recent calculated median eGFR was 57 $mL/min/1.73m^2$ for the entire cohort. Greater than 95% of subjects were able to avoid RRT. This work has demonstrated that at a minimum of 10 years after initial surgery and despite the need for repeat surgical interventions on the same kidney, NSS allows for excellent oncologic and functional outcomes in selected patients.

2.2 Laparoscopic partial nephrectomy

LPN has gained acceptance as the *de facto* standard treatment for renal cortical tumors less than 4cm in size, when technically feasible by this approach (Lane and Gill 2007; Gong et al. 2008; Lane and Gill 2010). Initially employed to resect small, exophytic renal masses, the indications have expanded to include completely endophytic tumors, hilar tumors and

tumors that measure 4–7cm in size (Gill et al. 2006; Permpongkosol et al. 2006; Lattouf et al. 2008; Simmons et al. 2009; Shikanov et al. 2010). The challenges of LPN, when compared to OPN, include completely resecting the tumor in a bloodless field and performing the necessary renorrhaphy while simultaneously minimizing warm ischemic time.
Several of these challenges have been overcome with technical modifications to the surgery including magnified visualization, improved tools for intracorporal suturing and cold ischemia, as well as improved laparoscopic equipment.

	Johnson et al. (2008)	Bratslavsky et al. (2008)
Partial Nephrectomy Type	Repeat	Salvage
Patients, *n*	47	11
Partial nephrectomy, *n*	51	13
Median tumors removed (range)	7 (1-55)	5 (1-27)
Median EBL, *mL* (range)	1,800 (50-21,500)	2,100 (200-12,000)
Transfusion Requirement (%)	38 (75)	10 (77)
Median Units Transfused (Range)	2 (0-31)	4.5 (0-18)
Intraoperative Complications		
Visceral or vascular injury (%)	2 (4)	6 (46)
Ureteral Injury (%)	1	0
Postoperative complications		
Prolonged Urine Leak (%)	8 (15)	2 (15)
Permanent Hemodialysis (%)	3 (6)	2 (15)
Renal Unit Loss (%)	3 (6)	3 (23)
Rhabdomyolysis (%)	0	1 (8)
Reoperation (%)	2 (4)	4 (36)
Cardiovascular events (%)	1 (2)	0

Table 2. Repeat and Salvage PN Outcomes

As urologists gained more experience with LPN, more centers have employed LPN for technically challenging scenarios where OPN was historically utilized. Tumors that are centrally located and close to the hilum mean the surgeon will encounter larger blood vessles and must perform a more extensive renorrhaphy, often with pelvicaliceal repair. Nadu and colleagues found that LPN for peripheral (n=159) vs. central (n=53) tumors had similar estimated blood loss (EBL) and operative times, whereas WIT was longer for central masses (37 vs. 28 min) (Nadu et al. 2009). Richstone and colleagues evaluated their results with LPN for hilar tumors in 18 patients and reported a mean operative time of 173 min, WIT of 29.4 min and median EBL of 394 ml (Richstone et al. 2008). In addition to tumors in difficult locations, PN in the obese patient population have been shown to have a higher rate of postoperative complications, such as cardiovascular events, wound infections, DVT and wound dehiscence. Romero and colleagues compared LPN (n=56) and OPN (n=28) in an obese cohort and demonstrated that the LPN group had shorter operative time, decreased EBL and fewer intraoperative and postoperative complications compared to those treated by OPN (Romero et al. 2008).

With regards to oncologic outcomes when compared with OPN, LPN has proven to have equivalent 5 year outcomes for T1a lesions in numerous single institution and multi-institutional studies (Porpiglia et al. 2005; Permpongkosol et al. 2006; Bollens et al. 2007; Gill et al. 2007; Lane and Gill 2007; Marszalek et al. 2009; Simmons et al. 2009). Rassweiler and colleagues reported a local recurrence rate of 1.41% among all the urologic malignancies treated in 1098 patients who underwent mixed urologic laparoscopic procedures over a ten year period with a median follow-up of 5 years (Rassweiler et al. 2003). More recently, the Cleveland Clinic reported 5 year survival data after LPN (n=58) with a mean follow-up of 5.7 years (Lane and Gill 2007). Overall survival was 86% and cancer specific survival was 100%. They did not report development of metastatic disease and documented a single local recurrence (2.7%). These findings were consistent with other reported cancer specific survival in reported LPN series which range from 91.4% to 100%.

The overall local recurrence rate in reported LPN series range from 0% to 2.4% with positive surgical margins ranging from 0% to 2.9% (Porpiglia et al. 2005; Lane and Gill 2007; Lane and Gill 2010). Simmons and colleagues reported on the eqiuivalence of oncologic outomes in select patients with clinical stage T1b–T3 tumors treated with LPN compared to a matched cohort of patients who underwent laparoscopic radical nephrectomy (Simmons et al. 2009). The cancer specific survival rate in both groups was 97% and the recurrence free survival was 97% and 94% in the laparoscopic radical nephrectomy and LPN groups, respectively. In a multi-institutional study, Porpiglia and colleagues described LPN for T1b masses in 63 patients and reported intraoperative hemorrhage in 7.3% of cases and postoperative complications in 14.6% of cases (Porpiglia et al. 2010). (Table 3)

Author (Year)	No. of patients	Mean tumor size (cm)	CSS (%)	Positive Surgical Margin (%)	Local recurrence (%)	Mean Follow-up (mo)
Bollens et al (2007)	39	2.3	100	2.6	0	15
Permpongkosol et al (2006)	85	2.4	97.6	2.4	1.7	40
Gill et al (2007)	771	2.7	99.3	1.6	1.4	14
Marszalek et al (2009)	100	2.8	96.3	4	3	44
Lane et al (2007)	58	2.9	100	1.7	1.7	68
Simmons et al (2009)	35	4.9	97	0	6	44
Porpiglia et al (2010)	63	4.7	N/A	6.5	0	N/A

Table 3. Oncologic Outcomes of Contemporary LPN Series

Although comparisons of open and laparoscopic PN have been performed, all studies are retrospective, and no randomized studies have been done so far. Nevertheless, the available literature suggests the equivalence of LPN to OPN for renal cortical tumors. Gill and colleagues in a multi-institutional study compared LPN (n=1029) and OPN (n=771) in 1800 patients with a renal cortical tumor measuring less than 7cm (Gill et al. 2007). In that study, patients undergoing OPN were a higher risk group with decreased performance status, renal functional impairment and more tumors greater than 4cm. The authors reported a positive surgical margin rate of 2.85% for LPN versus 1.26% for OPN and three year cancer specific survival of 99.3% for LPN and 99.2% for OPN. Marszalek and colleagues performed a matched-pair comparison of 200 patients matched for age, sex, and tumor size who underwent OPN (n=100) and LPN (n=100) with median 3.6 year follow-up (Marszalek et al. 2009). The stage of renal cell cancer was pT1 in all cases and the average tumor size was 2.8cm in the LPN cohort and 2.9cm in the OPN cohort. They reported a positive surgical margin rate of 4% and 2% in the LPN and OPN cohorts, respectively. Estimated 5 year local recurrence free survival using Kaplan-Meier method was 97% and 98%, and distant recurrence free survival was 99% and 96% in the LPN and OPN cohorts, respectively.

In summary, use of LPN has expanded from its initial use for the extirpation of smaller exophytic lesions to larger T1b tumors, endophytic and hilar lesions. It appears that for tumors less than 4cm in size, LPN provides equivalent oncologic control to OPN at intermediate follow-up. Oncologic outcomes are encouraging for tumors in the 4-7cm range although intermediate term oncologic data has yet to be reported.

2.3 Robotic assisted partial nephrectomy

With the establishment of LPN as an alternative to OPN in the treatment of renal cortical masses, RAPN has been increasingly adopted by urologic surgeons with the goal of broadening the utilization of NSS while still providing the advantages of minimally invasive surgery. Established advantages of minimally invasive techniques for PN include decreased postoperative pain, decreased hospital stay and shorter convalescence compared with standard open technique. This alternative to LPN may aid in the learning curve and facilitate in the reconstructive aspects of what is a technically demanding operation. Features of the robotic platform include stereoscopic vision, articulating instruments, and motion scaling to reduce tremor. These amenities may allow the surgeon to replicate established maneuvers employed during OPN, allow for extirpation of complex, centrally located tumors, and reconstruction of the pelvicaliceal system.

The feasibility and safety of RAPN has been demonstrated in several small, single institution studies (Gettman et al. 2004; Phillips et al. 2005; Caruso et al. 2006; Kaul et al. 2007; Aron et al. 2008; Deane et al. 2008; Benway et al. 2009; Ho et al. 2009; Michli and Parra 2009; Benway et al. 2010). Recent studies have demonstrated the feasibility of RAPN for larger, deeper tumors that are hilar in their location as well as for multiple tumors in the hereditary renal cancer population (Rogers et al. 2008; Boris et al. 2009; Gupta et al. 2011). (Table 4)

In a recent review of the RAPN literature, Shapiro and colleagues analyzed the results of the largest series of RAPN and reported an overall positive surgical margin rate of 3.3% (7/211) and that at up to 54 months of follow-up, there were no local or distant recurrences (Shapiro et al. 2009). With the expansion of LPN to T1b tumors, RAPN has also been employed for these challenging tumors. Patel and colleagues retrospectively analyzed a cohort of 71 patients who underwent RAPN for tumors greater than 4cm (n=15) compared to those with tumors less than 4cm (N=56) (Patel et al. 2010). There were no positive surgical margins in the greater than 4cm group and 3 reported in the less than 4 cm group for an overall rate of 5.4% but the authors noted that on final pathology only 1 of the positive surgical margins was for a malignancy with no sequelae at one year. Gupta and colleagues reported on 19 surgeries for multiple tumors (average 2.3 tumors/kidney) with the largest tumor greater than 4cm (Gupta et al. 2010). Remarkably, in this population, no patient required a blood transfusion and mean WIT was 36 min. There are currently no intermediate or long term oncologic outcomes reported in the literature for RAPN, but short term outcomes from several robotic series seem to be equivalent to those reported for LPN series. However, these data are immature at best and long term data is needed regarding oncologic outcomes.

Author (Year)	No. of RAPN	Mean tumor size (cm)	Mean WIT (min)	Mean operative time (min)	Mean blood-loss (ml)	Positive surgical margin	Mean Follow-up (mo)
Boris et al (2009)	10	2.3 (multiple)	29.6	257	360	not assessed	9
Scoll et al (2010)	98	2.8	25.5	203	127	5	13
Rogers et al (2008)	148	2.8	27.8	197	183	6	7
Benway et al (2010)	183	2.9	23.9	210	131.5	4	16
Rogers et al 2008)	8	3.6	31	192	230	0	3
Patel et al (2010)	15	5	25	275	100	0	7
Gupta et al (2010)	19	5 (multiple)	36	390	500	not assessed	22

Table 4. Selected RAPN Series

3. Renal functional outcomes

While it is intuitive that sparing normal renal parenchyma will impart better overall kidney function, the misconception long held is that the sacrifice of normal functioning nephrons via radical nephrectomy will not cause serious long term side effects. However, one of the most important recent concepts to be recognized is the adverse effects of renal insufficiency on compounding medical comorbidities. Although no randomized prospective studies exist at this time, retrospective analysis revealed that incremental increases in renal insufficiency are associated with incremental increases in all-cause hospitalization, cardiovascular morbidity and all-cause mortality (Go et al. 2004). Additionally, several other studies demonstrated a close association of renal insufficiency with cardiovascular disease, while others have suggested that patients treated with radical nephrectomy had shorter overall survival when compared to those treated with PN (Russo and Huang 2008; Huang et al. 2009). Two studies comparing late renal functional outcomes in over 450 patients undergoing radical nephrectomy and PN demonstrated that patients undergoing radical nephrectomy were more likely to have serum creatinine levels elevated to more than 2.0 mg/dL and proteinuria (Lau et al. 2000). A more recent study from the Mayo Clinic identified 648 patients treated with radical nephrectomy or PN for tumors less than or equal to 4 cm and a normal contralateral kidney (Thompson et al. 2008). Overall survival calculated in 327 patients under the age of 65 after controlling for year of surgery, diabetes at presentation, Charlson comorbidity score and tumor histology found that radical nephrectomy was significantly associated with an increased risk of death. These results strongly indicate that the use of radical nephrectomy for small renal masses is unjustified oncologically and that NSS should be selected whenever possible.

Duration and type of "safe" ischemia has been actively evaluated in recent years. A large multi-institutional study evaluated the effects of ischemic time on renal function in patients undergoing OPN without ischemia, with warm ischemia, and with cold ischemia. This study included patients with solitary kidneys and defined chronic renal insufficiency on the basis of serum creatinine. The conclusion of this study was that WIT should be limited to 20 minutes and cold ischemia time to less than 35 minutes to avoid an increased risk of chronic renal insufficiency and acute renal failure (Simmons et al. 2008; Becker et al. 2009). As the urologic community has gained experience with LPN and RAPN, WIT has been reduced and in several studies it was found comparable to that of OPN. (Table 4) Regardless, until prospective data can determine the true safe maximum WIT in regards to renal function, every attempt to minimize WIT should be made.

4. Future directions for partial nephrectomy

With the establishment that PN for renal tumors up to 7cm is oncologically equivalent to radical nephrectomy, urologic oncologists have been expanding the indications for PN to include tumors greater than 7cm (T2) and even lesions that penetrate the renal capsule (T3a) or have tumor thrombus involving the main renal vein (T3b). Breau and colleagues from the Mayo Clinic recently reported their experience treating 69 subjects with advanced renal tumors (T2=32, T3a=28, T3b=9) who were compared to a matched cohort from their kidney tumor registry (Breau et al. 2010). Cancer-specific and overall death rates were similar between the two groups ($p=0.489$ and $p=0.642$, respectively), and differences in metastatic disease and local recurrence at an average follow-up of 3.2 years were not statistically significant ($p=0.92$ and 0.234, respectively). Renal function, however, as measured by serum creatinine, was better preserved in the PN group (9.5% increase vs. 33% increase; $p<0.001$).

Similarly, several small series have been reported in which NSS was used in the cytoreductive setting for patients with metastatic disease (Krambeck et al. 2006; Hutterer et al. 2007). The majority of these cases were performed on solitary kidneys or in the presence of renal insufficiency. Survival was not negatively impacted when compared to historic controls who received radical nephrectomy, and renal function was preserved adequately to avoid RRT, which will help facilitate access to targeted systemic treatments (Singer et al. 2010; Singer et al. 2011). Targeted systemic therapy has also been used in the neoadjuvant setting to downsize the primary tumor in a solitary kidney so that PN would be technically feasible (Shuch et al. 2008).

In the years ahead, it is unlikely that tumor diameter will be a major determinant for the type of renal surgery offered to a patient with a renal mass. Instead of size, the surgeon will base his or her recommendation for or against NSS on objective measures of the feasibility of a safe and complete resection (Lane et al. 2010). Most recently, Bratslavsky has raised the concept of the metastatic potential of renal tumors, in which the development of metastatic disease is not prevented by removal of the normal renal parenchyma. He argues against arbitrary size cut-offs traditionally used for selection of patients for partial nephrectomy, and suggests that maximal preservation of normal parenchyma in patients with largest tumors may be even more important, as these patients would be at a higher risk for metastatic disease and could benefit for future adjuvant trials or treatment (Bratslavsky, 2011). Finally, as urologists continue to report and compare their NSS outcomes, they will need to use a new metric, such as the RENAL nephrometry score or the PADUA classification, which objectively quantifies the anatomic complexity of a renal mass (Kutikov and Uzzo 2009; Ficarra et al. 2009).

5. Conclusions

NSS should be considered the preferred therapy for renal tumors whenever it is technically feasible via any surgical approach. Patients and their referring physicians should seek out high-volume centers and experienced surgeons who have a special interest in NSS. The method of PN selected, whether OPN, LPN, or RAPN, matters far less than ensuring that the correct operation is performed for the appropriate indications. Since the loss of renal function can increase the risk of post-operative morbidity and mortality in numerous ways, PN must continue to be the treatment of choice for kidney tumors. PN is the oncologically sound and functionally prudent way to manage an increasing number of renal tumors.

6. Acknowledgement

This research was supported by the Intramural Research Program of the NIH, National Cancer Institute, Center for Cancer Research.

7. References

Ansari, M.S., Gupta, N.P.& Kumar, P. (2003). "von Hippel-Lindau disease with bilateral multiple renal cell carcinoma managed by right radical nephrectomy and left repeat partial nephrectomy." *Int Urol Nephrol* 35(4): 471-473.

Aron, M., Koenig, P., Kaouk, J.H., Nguyen, M.M., Desai, M.M.& Gill, I.S. (2008). "Robotic and laparoscopic partial nephrectomy: a matched-pair comparison from a high-volume centre." *BJU Int* 102(1): 86-92.

Becker, F., Siemer, S., Hack, M., Humke, U., Ziegler, M.& Stockle, M. (2006). "Excellent long-term cancer control with elective nephron-sparing surgery for selected renal cell carcinomas measuring more than 4 cm." *Eur Urol* 49(6): 1058-1063; discussion 1063-1054.

Becker, F., Siemer, S., Humke, U., Hack, M., Ziegler, M.& Stockle, M. (2006). "Elective nephron sparing surgery should become standard treatment for small unilateral renal cell carcinoma: Long-term survival data of 216 patients." *Eur Urol* 49(2): 308-313.

Becker, F., Van Poppel, H., Hakenberg, O.W., Stief, C., Gill, I., Guazzoni, G., Montorsi, F., Russo, P.& Stockle, M. (2009). "Assessing the impact of ischaemia time during partial nephrectomy." *Eur Urol* 56(4): 625-634.

Belldegrun, A.S., Klatte, T., Shuch, B., LaRochelle, J.C., Miller, D.C., Said, J.W., Riggs, S.B., Zomorodian, N., Kabbinavar, F.F., Dekernion, J.B.& Pantuck, A.J. (2008). "Cancer-specific survival outcomes among patients treated during the cytokine era of kidney cancer (1989-2005): a benchmark for emerging targeted cancer therapies." *Cancer* 113(9): 2457-2463.

Benway, B.M., Bhayani, S.B., Rogers, C.G., Porter, J.R., Buffi, N.M., Figenshau, R.S.& Mottrie, A. (2010). "Robot-assisted partial nephrectomy: an international experience." *Eur Urol* 57(5): 815-820.

Benway, B.M., Wang, A.J., Cabello, J.M.& Bhayani, S.B. (2009). "Robotic partial nephrectomy with sliding-clip renorrhaphy: technique and outcomes." *Eur Urol* 55(3): 592-599.

Bollens, R., Rosenblatt, A., Espinoza, B.P., De Groote, A., Quackels, T., Roumeguere, T., Vanden Bossche, M., Wespes, E., Zlotta, A.R.& Schulman, C.C. (2007). "Laparoscopic partial nephrectomy with "on-demand" clamping reduces warm ischemia time." *Eur Urol* 52(3): 804-809.

Boris, R., Proano, M., Linehan, W.M., Pinto, P.A.& Bratslavsky, G. (2009). "Initial experience with robot assisted partial nephrectomy for multiple renal masses." *J Urol* 182(4): 1280-1286.

Bratslavsky, G., Liu, J.J., Johnson, A.D., Sudarshan, S., Choyke, P.L., Linehan, W.M.& Pinto, P.A. (2008). "Salvage partial nephrectomy for hereditary renal cancer: feasibility and outcomes." *J Urol* 179(1): 67-70.

Bratslavsky, G. (2011) "Argument in favor of performing partial nephrectomy for tumors greater than 7cm: The metastatic prescription has already been written." *Urol Oncol* 29(6):892-32.

Breau, R.H., Crispen, P.L., Jimenez, R.E., Lohse, C.M., Blute, M.L.& Leibovich, B.C. (2010). "Outcome of stage T2 or greater renal cell cancer treated with partial nephrectomy." *J Urol* 183(3): 903-908.

Campbell, S.C., Novick, A.C., Belldegrun, A., Blute, M.L., Chow, G.K., Derweesh, I.H., Faraday, M.M., Kaouk, J.H., Leveillee, R.J., Matin, S.F., Russo, P.& Uzzo, R.G. (2009). "Guideline for management of the clinical T1 renal mass." *J Urol* 182(4): 1271-1279.

Carini, M., Minervini, A., Lapini, A., Masieri, L.& Serni, S. (2006). "Simple enucleation for the treatment of renal cell carcinoma between 4 and 7 cm in greatest dimension: progression and long-term survival." *J Urol* 175(6): 2022-2026; discussion 2026.

Carini, M., Minervini, A., Masieri, L., Lapini, A.& Serni, S. (2006). "Simple enucleation for the treatment of PT1a renal cell carcinoma: our 20-year experience." *Eur Urol* 50(6): 1263-1268; discussion 1269-1271.

Caruso, R.P., Phillips, C.K., Kau, E., Taneja, S.S.& Stifelman, M.D. (2006). "Robot assisted laparoscopic partial nephrectomy: initial experience." *J Urol* 176(1): 36-39.

Chow, W.H., Devesa, S.S., Warren, J.L.& Fraumeni, J.F., Jr. (1999). "Rising incidence of renal cell cancer in the United States." *JAMA* 281(17): 1628-1631.

Dash, A., Vickers, A.J., Schachter, L.R., Bach, A.M., Snyder, M.E.& Russo, P. (2006). "Comparison of outcomes in elective partial vs radical nephrectomy for clear cell renal cell carcinoma of 4-7 cm." *BJU Int* 97(5): 939-945.

Deane, L.A., Lee, H.J., Box, G.N., Melamud, O., Yee, D.S., Abraham, J.B., Finley, D.S., Borin, J.F., McDougall, E.M., Clayman, R.V.& Ornstein, D.K. (2008). "Robotic versus standard laparoscopic partial/wedge nephrectomy: a comparison of intraoperative and perioperative results from a single institution." *J Endourol* 22(5): 947-952.

Duffey, B.G., Choyke, P.L., Glenn, G., Grubb, R.L., Venzon, D., Linehan, W.M.& Walther, M.M. (2004). "The relationship between renal tumor size and metastases in patients with von Hippel-Lindau disease." *J Urol* 172(1): 63-65.

Fergany, A.F., Saad, I.R., Woo, L.& Novick, A.C. (2006). "Open partial nephrectomy for tumor in a solitary kidney: experience with 400 cases." *J Urol* 175(5): 1630-1633; discussion 1633.

Ficarra, V., Novara, G., Secco, S., Macchi, V., Porzionato, A., De Caro, R.& Artibani, W. (2009). "Preoperative aspects and dimensions used for an anatomical (PADUA) classification of renal tumours in patients who are candidates for nephron-sparing surgery." *Eur Urol* 56(5): 786-793.

Gettman, M.T., Blute, M.L., Chow, G.K., Neururer, R., Bartsch, G.& Peschel, R. (2004). "Robotic-assisted laparoscopic partial nephrectomy: technique and initial clinical experience with DaVinci robotic system." *Urology* 64(5): 914-918.

Gill, I.S., Colombo, J.R., Jr., Moinzadeh, A., Finelli, A., Ukimura, O., Tucker, K., Kaouk, J.& Desai, M. (2006). "Laparoscopic partial nephrectomy in solitary kidney." *J Urol* 175(2): 454-458.

Gill, I.S., Kavoussi, L.R., Lane, B.R., Blute, M.L., Babineau, D., Colombo, J.R., Jr., Frank, I., Permpongkosol, S., Weight, C.J., Kaouk, J.H., Kattan, M.W.& Novick, A.C. (2007). "Comparison of 1,800 laparoscopic and open partial nephrectomies for single renal tumors." *J Urol* 178(1): 41-46.

Go, A.S., Chertow, G.M., Fan, D., McCulloch, C.E.& Hsu, C.Y. (2004). "Chronic kidney disease and the risks of death, cardiovascular events, and hospitalization." *N Engl J Med* 351(13): 1296-1305.

Gong, E.M., Orvieto, M.A., Zorn, K.C., Lucioni, A., Steinberg, G.D.& Shalhav, A.L. (2008). "Comparison of laparoscopic and open partial nephrectomy in clinical T1a renal tumors." *J Endourol* 22(5): 953-957.

Gupta, G.N., Boris, R., Chung, P., Marston Linehan, W., Pinto, P.A.& Bratslavsky, G. (2011). "Robot-assisted laparoscopic partial nephrectomy for tumors greater than 4 cm and high nephrometry score: Feasibility, renal functional, and oncological outcomes with minimum 1 year follow-up." *Urol Oncol.*

Ho, H., Schwentner, C., Neururer, R., Steiner, H., Bartsch, G.& Peschel, R. (2009). "Robotic-assisted laparoscopic partial nephrectomy: surgical technique and clinical outcomes at 1 year." *BJU Int* 103(5): 663-668.

Hock, L.M., Lynch, J.& Balaji, K.C. (2002). "Increasing incidence of all stages of kidney cancer in the last 2 decades in the United States: an analysis of surveillance, epidemiology and end results program data." *J Urol* 167(1): 57-60.

Huang, W.C., Elkin, E.B., Levey, A.S., Jang, T.L.& Russo, P. (2009). "Partial nephrectomy versus radical nephrectomy in patients with small renal tumors--is there a difference in mortality and cardiovascular outcomes?" *J Urol* 181(1): 55-61; discussion 61-52.

Hutterer, G.C., Patard, J.J., Colombel, M., Belldegrun, A.S., Pfister, C., Guille, F., Artibani, W., Montorsi, F., Pantuck, A.J.& Karakiewicz, P.I. (2007). "Cytoreductive nephron-sparing surgery does not appear to undermine disease-specific survival in patients with metastatic renal cell carcinoma." *Cancer* 110(11): 2428-2433.

Jemal, A., Bray, F., Center, M.M., Ferlay, J., Ward, E.& Forman, D. (2011). "Global cancer statistics." *CA Cancer J Clin.*

Jemal, A., Siegel, R., Xu, J.& Ward, E. (2010). "Cancer statistics, 2010." *CA Cancer J Clin* 60(5): 277-300.

Johnson, A., Sudarshan, S., Liu, J., Linehan, W.M., Pinto, P.A.& Bratslavsky, G. (2008). "Feasibility and outcomes of repeat partial nephrectomy." *J Urol* 180(1): 89-93; discussion 93.

Kaul, S., Laungani, R., Sarle, R., Stricker, H., Peabody, J., Littleton, R.& Menon, M. (2007). "da Vinci-assisted robotic partial nephrectomy: technique and results at a mean of 15 months of follow-up." *Eur Urol* 51(1): 186-191; discussion 191-182.

Krambeck, A.E., Leibovich, B.C., Lohse, C.M., Kwon, E.D., Zincke, H.& Blute, M.L. (2006). "The role of nephron sparing surgery for metastatic (pM1) renal cell carcinoma." *J Urol* 176(5): 1990-1995; discussion 1995.

Kutikov, A.& Uzzo, R.G. (2009). "The R.E.N.A.L. nephrometry score: a comprehensive standardized system for quantitating renal tumor size, location and depth." *J Urol* 182(3): 844-853.

Lane, B.R., Fergany, A.F., Linehan, W.M.& Bratslavsky, G. (2010). "Should preservable parenchyma, and not tumor size, be the main determinant of the feasibility of partial nephrectomy?" *Urology* 76(3): 608-609.

Lane, B.R.& Gill, I.S. (2007). "5-Year outcomes of laparoscopic partial nephrectomy." *J Urol* 177(1): 70-74; discussion 74.

Lane, B.R.& Gill, I.S. (2010). "7-year oncological outcomes after laparoscopic and open partial nephrectomy." *J Urol* 183(2): 473-479.

Lattouf, J.B., Beri, A., D'Ambros, O.F., Grull, M., Leeb, K.& Janetschek, G. (2008). "Laparoscopic partial nephrectomy for hilar tumors: technique and results." *Eur Urol* 54(2): 409-416.

Lau, W.K., Blute, M.L., Weaver, A.L., Torres, V.E.& Zincke, H. (2000). "Matched comparison of radical nephrectomy vs nephron-sparing surgery in patients with unilateral renal cell carcinoma and a normal contralateral kidney." *Mayo Clin Proc* 75(12): 1236-1242.

Leibovich, B.C., Blute, M.L., Cheville, J.C., Lohse, C.M., Weaver, A.L.& Zincke, H. (2004). "Nephron sparing surgery for appropriately selected renal cell carcinoma between 4 and 7 cm results in outcome similar to radical nephrectomy." *J Urol* 171(3): 1066-1070.

Ljungberg, B., Cowan, N.C., Hanbury, D.C., Hora, M., Kuczyk, M.A., Merseburger, A.S., Patard, J.J., Mulders, P.F.& Sinescu, I.C. (2010). "EAU guidelines on renal cell carcinoma: the 2010 update." *Eur Urol* 58(3): 398-406.

Margreiter, M.& Marberger, M. (2010). "Current status of open partial nephrectomy." *Curr Opin Urol* 20(5): 361-364.

Marszalek, M., Meixl, H., Polajnar, M., Rauchenwald, M., Jeschke, K.& Madersbacher, S. (2009). "Laparoscopic and open partial nephrectomy: a matched-pair comparison of 200 patients." *Eur Urol* 55(5): 1171-1178.

Michli, E.E.& Parra, R.O. (2009). "Robotic-assisted laparoscopic partial nephrectomy: initial clinical experience." *Urology* 73(2): 302-305.

Minervini, A., Ficarra, V., Rocco, F., Antonelli, A., Bertini, R., Carmignani, G., Cosciani Cunico, S., Fontana, D., Longo, N., Martorana, G., Mirone, V., Morgia, G., Novara, G., Roscigno, M., Schiavina, R., Serni, S., Simeone, C., Simonato, A., Siracusano, S., Volpe, A., Zattoni, F., Zucchi, A.& Carini, M. (2011). "Simple enucleation is equivalent to traditional partial nephrectomy for renal cell carcinoma: results of a nonrandomized, retrospective, comparative study." *J Urol* 185(5): 1604-1610.

Nadu, A., Kleinmann, N., Laufer, M., Dotan, Z., Winkler, H.& Ramon, J. (2009). "Laparoscopic partial nephrectomy for central tumors: analysis of perioperative outcomes and complications." *J Urol* 181(1): 42-47; discussion 47.

Novick, A.C.& Streem, S.B. (1992). "Long-term followup after nephron sparing surgery for renal cell carcinoma in von Hippel-Lindau disease." *J Urol* 147(6): 1488-1490.

Pahernik, S., Roos, F., Hampel, C., Gillitzer, R., Melchior, S.W.& Thuroff, J.W. (2006). "Nephron sparing surgery for renal cell carcinoma with normal contralateral kidney: 25 years of experience." *J Urol* 175(6): 2027-2031.

Patard, J.J., Shvarts, O., Lam, J.S., Pantuck, A.J., Kim, H.L., Ficarra, V., Cindolo, L., Han, K.R., De La Taille, A., Tostain, J., Artibani, W., Abbou, C.C., Lobel, B., Chopin, D.K., Figlin, R.A., Mulders, P.F.& Belldegrun, A.S. (2004). "Safety and efficacy of partial nephrectomy for all T1 tumors based on an international multicenter experience." *J Urol* 171(6 Pt 1): 2181-2185, quiz 2435.

Patel, M.N., Krane, L.S., Bhandari, A., Laungani, R.G., Shrivastava, A., Siddiqui, S.A., Menon, M.& Rogers, C.G. (2010). "Robotic partial nephrectomy for renal tumors larger than 4 cm." *Eur Urol* 57(2): 310-316.

Permpongkosol, S., Bagga, H.S., Romero, F.R., Sroka, M., Jarrett, T.W.& Kavoussi, L.R. (2006). "Laparoscopic versus open partial nephrectomy for the treatment of pathological T1N0M0 renal cell carcinoma: a 5-year survival rate." *J Urol* 176(5): 1984-1988; discussion 1988-1989.

Phillips, C.K., Taneja, S.S.& Stifelman, M.D. (2005). "Robot-assisted laparoscopic partial nephrectomy: the NYU technique." *J Endourol* 19(4): 441-445; discussion 445.

Porpiglia, F., Fiori, C., Piechaud, T., Gaston, R., Guazzoni, G., Pansadoro, V., Bachmann, A.& Janetschek, G. (2010). "Laparoscopic partial nephrectomy for large renal masses: results of a European survey." *World J Urol* 28(4): 525-529.

Porpiglia, F., Fiori, C., Terrone, C., Bollito, E., Fontana, D.& Scarpa, R.M. (2005). "Assessment of surgical margins in renal cell carcinoma after nephron sparing: a comparative study: laparoscopy vs open surgery." *J Urol* 173(4): 1098-1101.

Rassweiler, J., Tsivian, A., Kumar, A.V., Lymberakis, C., Schulze, M., Seeman, O.& Frede, T. (2003). "Oncological safety of laparoscopic surgery for urological malignancy: experience with more than 1,000 operations." *J Urol* 169(6): 2072-2075.

Richstone, L., Montag, S., Ost, M., Reggio, E., Permpongkosol, S.& Kavoussi, L.R. (2008). "Laparoscopic partial nephrectomy for hilar tumors: evaluation of short-term oncologic outcome." *Urology* 71(1): 36-40.

Rini, B.I. (2009). "Metastatic renal cell carcinoma: many treatment options, one patient." *J Clin Oncol* 27(19): 3225-3234.

Rogers, C.G., Singh, A., Blatt, A.M., Linehan, W.M.& Pinto, P.A. (2008). "Robotic partial nephrectomy for complex renal tumors: surgical technique." *Eur Urol* 53(3): 514-521.

Romero, F.R., Rais-Bahrami, S., Muntener, M., Brito, F.A., Jarrett, T.W.& Kavoussi, L.R. (2008). "Laparoscopic partial nephrectomy in obese and non-obese patients: comparison with open surgery." *Urology* 71(5): 806-809.

Russo, P. (2007). "Open partial nephrectomy: an essential operation with an expanding role." *Curr Opin Urol* 17(5): 309-315.

Russo, P., Goetzl, M., Simmons, R., Katz, J., Motzer, R.& Reuter, V. (2002). "Partial nephrectomy: the rationale for expanding the indications." *Ann Surg Oncol* 9(7): 680-687.

Russo, P.& Huang, W. (2008). "The medical and oncological rationale for partial nephrectomy for the treatment of T1 renal cortical tumors." *Urol Clin North Am* 35(4): 635-643; vii.

Shapiro, E., Benway, B.M., Wang, A.J.& Bhayani, S.B. (2009). "The role of nephron-sparing robotic surgery in the management of renal malignancy." *Curr Opin Urol* 19(1): 76-80.

Shikanov, S., Lifshitz, D.A., Deklaj, T., Katz, M.H.& Shalhav, A.L. (2010). "Laparoscopic partial nephrectomy for technically challenging tumours." *BJU Int* 106(1): 91-94.

Shuch, B., Riggs, S.B., LaRochelle, J.C., Kabbinavar, F.F., Avakian, R., Pantuck, A.J., Patard, J.J.& Belldegrun, A.S. (2008). "Neoadjuvant targeted therapy and advanced kidney cancer: observations and implications for a new treatment paradigm." *BJU Int* 102(6): 692-696.

Simmons, M.N., Schreiber, M.J.& Gill, I.S. (2008). "Surgical renal ischemia: a contemporary overview." *J Urol* 180(1): 19-30.

Simmons, M.N., Weight, C.J.& Gill, I.S. (2009). "Laparoscopic radical versus partial nephrectomy for tumors >4 cm: intermediate-term oncologic and functional outcomes." *Urology* 73(5): 1077-1082.

Singer, E.A.& Bratslavsky, G. (2010). "Management of locally recurrent kidney cancer." *Curr Urol Rep* 11(1): 15-21.

Singer, E.A., Bratslavsky, G., Linehan, W.M.& Srinivasan, R. (2010). "Targeted therapies for non-clear renal cell carcinoma." *Target Oncol* 5(2): 119-129.

Singer, E.A., Gupta, G.N.& Srinivasan, R. (2011). "Update on targeted therapies for clear cell renal cell carcinoma." *Curr Opin Oncol* 23(3): 283-289.

Singer, E.A., Vourganti, S., Lin, K., Rastinehad, A., Pinto, P.A., Gupta, G.N., Linehan, W.M.& Bratslavsky, G. (2011). "Outcomes of Patients with Surgically Treated Bilateral Renal Masses and a Minimum of 10 Years of Follow-Up: The NCI Experience." *J Urol* 185(4 Supp): e746.

Steinbach, F., Novick, A.C., Zincke, H., Miller, D.P., Williams, R.D., Lund, G., Skinner, D.G., Esrig, D., Richie, J.P., deKernion, J.B.& et al. (1995). "Treatment of renal cell carcinoma in von Hippel-Lindau disease: a multicenter study." *J Urol* 153(6): 1812-1816.

Sutherland, S.E., Resnick, M.I., Maclennan, G.T.& Goldman, H.B. (2002). "Does the size of the surgical margin in partial nephrectomy for renal cell cancer really matter?" *J Urol* 167(1): 61-64.

Thompson, R.H., Boorjian, S.A., Lohse, C.M., Leibovich, B.C., Kwon, E.D., Cheville, J.C.& Blute, M.L. (2008). "Radical nephrectomy for pT1a renal masses may be associated with decreased overall survival compared with partial nephrectomy." *J Urol* 179(2): 468-471; discussion 472-463.

Van Poppel, H., Da Pozzo, L., Albrecht, W., Matveev, V., Bono, A., Borkowski, A., Colombel, M., Klotz, L., Skinner, E., Keane, T., Marreaud, S., Collette, S.& Sylvester, R. (2011).

"A prospective, randomised EORTC intergroup phase 3 study comparing the oncologic outcome of elective nephron-sparing surgery and radical nephrectomy for low-stage renal cell carcinoma." *Eur Urol* 59(4): 543-552.

Volpe, A., Cadeddu, J.A., Cestari, A., Gill, I.S., Jewett, M.A., Joniau, S., Kirkali, Z., Marberger, M., Patard, J.J., Staehler, M.& Uzzo, R.G. (2011). "Contemporary management of small renal masses." *Eur Urol* 60(3): 501-515.

Walther, M.M., Choyke, P.L., Glenn, G., Lyne, J.C., Rayford, W., Venzon, D.& Linehan, W.M. (1999). "Renal cancer in families with hereditary renal cancer: prospective analysis of a tumor size threshold for renal parenchymal sparing surgery." *J Urol* 161(5): 1475-1479.

5

Image-Guided Percutaneous Ablation of Renal Tumors

Majid Maybody, Joseph P. Erinjeri and Stephen B. Solomon
Memorial Sloan-Kettering Cancer Center New York,
New York
U.S.A.

1. Introduction

Renal tumors account for more than 50,000 new cases annually in the United States with a rising incidence (Chow et al., 1999). This is mainly because of an increase in diagnosis due to widespread use of cross-sectional imaging (Pantuck et al., 2001). Renal cell carcinoma constitutes 4% of all adult malignancies (American Cancer Society, 2008) and about 70 to 80 percent of patients presenting with localized limited-stage disease (Luciani et al., 2000; Janzen et al.,2003). Nephron-sparing surgery remians the gold standard treatment for small renal tumors. Although operative resection has been shown to be effective for treatment of small renal tumors and for preservation of renal function, it does have morbidity and mortality risks (Fergany et al., 2000; Gill et al., 2007; Breda et al., 2009). Early laparoscopic renal cryoablation results have shown technical feasibility and offer a less invasive technique for destroying small renal tumors (Spaliviero et al., 2004). Image-guided percutaneous ablation of small renal tumors is less invasive, incurs less damage to uninvolved noncancerous renal tissue and is becoming a viable alternative to nephron-sparing surgery (Hui et al., 2008, Gontero et al., 2010).

2. General concepts of percutaneous image-guided ablation

Ablation refers to the destruction of tissue in its original location without the removal of the treated tissue. A resection refers to the removal of tissues from the body. Cross-sectional imaging modalities enable the operator to safely target the tumor through the skin without the need for incisions (percutaneous). The most common imaging guidance modalities are ultrasound, computed tomography (CT), and magnetic resonance imaging (MRI). Energy is applied to the tumor via placement of needle-like devices called probes or applicators. The energy deposition results in irreversible damage to the tissues in its field; this area is called the ablation zone. Ablation procedures are usually performed by interventional radiologists and/or urologists (the operating physician). It can be performed in an outpatient setting. The most important factors in determining the outcome of an ablation are tumor size and location of tumor within the kidney. The best results are achieved in tumors less than 4 cm in diameter (Boss et al., 2005; Miki et al., 2006). The least challenging tumor location is posterior exophytic and the most challenging locations are central hilar and anterior. Central tumors carry a higher risk for bleeding, a higher risk of damage to hilar structures such as collecting system and vessels, and have a higher recurrence rate due to thermal sink effect. The thermal sink effect refers to the phenomenon whereby the thermal energy deposition to a tumor during ablation is dissipated by the blood flow in the vessels abutting the tumor. Depending on the location of an anterior tumor, it may be approachable percutaneously. However, treatment of these tumors may require a trans-renal or trans-hepatic approach. All tumors less than 3 cm can be treated in one session and the need for more than one ablation session increases with tumor size larger than 3 cm (Boss et al., 2005). Ablation of a 5 to 10 mm margin around the tumor is ideal to minimize the risk of recurrence.

3. Ablation modalities

The choice of percutaneous ablation modality is based on the availability of equipment, the operating physician's experience with a particular device and limitations based on anatomy and patient body habitus.

3.1 Radiofrequency ablation and cryoablation

Radiofrequency ablation (RFA) and cryoablation are the two most commonly used ablation modalities (Gervais et al., 2000; Joniau et al., 2010; Atwell et al., 2008). RFA destroys tumors by denaturing and hydrolyzing tumor proteins by heating them to temperatures above 60°C, whereas cryoablation destroys tumors by the formation of intracellular ice crystals which disrupt cell membranes by cooling them to temperatures generally below -20°C. Pathologically, both processes result in coagulation necrosis in the center and apoptosis in periphery of the treated tissues. , Both modalities are minimally invasive, as the thermal energy is applied by placing one or more probes into tumors. Each has unique technical features, and neither of the two has clearly been proven to be superior to the other (Maybody & Solomon, 2007; Mouraviev et al., 2007)(Table 1).

Radiofrequency Ablation	**Cryoablation**
Typical ablation: 20-30 minutes	Typical ablation: 30-40 minutes
Less bleeding	More bleeding
More pain (greater need for general anesthesia)	Less pain (moderate sedation)
Ablation zone not visible during ablation • Higher recurrence rates • Higher likelihood of repeat ablation	Ablation zone visible during ablation • Lower recurrence rates • Lower likelihood of repeat ablation
Larger ablation zone per applicator (requires fewer applicators)	Smaller ablation zone per applicator (requires more applicators)
CT monitoring during ablation difficult (artifacts)	CT monitoring during ablation possible
Interferes with pacemakers	No interference with pacemakers
More likely to damage the collecting system	Less likely to damage the collecting system (Janzen et al. 2005)
Less control over individual applicators	More control over individual applicators
Grounding pads (risk of skin burn)	Cumbersome equipment

Table 1. Comparison of main technical features of radiofrequency ablation and cryoablation in percutaneous image-guided ablation of renal tumors

3.2 Other ablation modalities

Microwave is a heat-based modality which involves deploying microwave energy (300-3000 MHz) from a non-tined probe (antenna) into a tumor causing oscillation of ions. This creates heat resulting in coagulative necrosis. Advantages include faster ablation times and less susceptibility to thermal heat-sink effect (Simon et al., 2005).

Laser is another heat-based ablation modality that deposits laser energy into the tumor via tiny flexible fiber optic conduits. Laser energy raises the tissue temperature and causes coagulative necrosis. Laser ablation has been successfully performed in renal tumors (Dick et al., 2002), and can be done under CT or MRI guidance. The flexibility of the fiber outside of the patient is an advantage when working in a CT or MRI gantry. Relative small ablation zones mandate multiple probe placements with laser ablation.

Irreversible electroporation (IRE) is a non-thermal ablation modality that causes apoptotic cell death by creating permanent microscopic pores in cell membranes when cells are exposed to specific electrical fields. This modality is much faster than other minimally invasive ablation techniques. Another advantage of IRE is that it is not affected by thermal sink phenomenon (Rubinsky et al., 2007). Preliminary animal and human experience is promising (Deodhar et al., 2011). Due to the stimulation of skeletal muscle by the electric field in IRE, the need for general anesthesia with paralytic agents remains a challenge to widespread use of the technique.

High-intensity focused ultrasound (HIFU) is a noninvasive heat-based ablation modality. It causes coagulation necrosis by focusing a high-intensity ultrasonic beam onto a small volume of target lesion. Respiratory movements and overlying ribs are major problems with the use of HIFU in renal tumors (Marberger et al., 2005; Klatte et al., 2009).

4. Imaging guidance

Percutaneous image-guided ablation can be performed under ultrasound, computed tomography (CT), or magnetic resonance imaging (MRI) guidance. The tumor should be well visualized on the imaging modality planned for the procedure. The advantages of ultrasound are its "real-time" capability and lack of ionizing radiation. Ultrasound can be used for accurate placement of probes before switching to CT or MRI for further monitoring. However, imaging with ultrasound is highly operator dependent and may be compromised in certain settings, such as patients with a large body habitus, the presence of abundant bowel gas, and when the tumor is near a focal loop of bowel that needs to be avoided. Another setback to ultrasound is the degradation of landmarks during ablation. In cryoablation, image degradation is caused by acoustic shadowing on the far side of the ice ball, and in RFA it is produced by micro bubbles.

CT is the most commonly used imaging modality for guidance (figure 1). It is not as operator dependent as ultrasound and is widely accessible to most operators. Its wide field of view is excellent to cover the critical organs and structures that need to be avoided. CT scanning is much less sensitive to body habitus than is ultrasound and CT images are not affected by bowel gas. If CT is chosen as image guidance method, the target lesion should ideally be visible on a non-contrast examination. Percutaneous ablation can be performed using a conventional CT scanner or a CT scanner with real-time fluoroscopic capability. Imaging monitoring with CT during active ablation with RFA is prone to significant artifacts due to interference of RF energy with the CT scanner. Cryoablation can be monitored by CT imaging during active ablation.

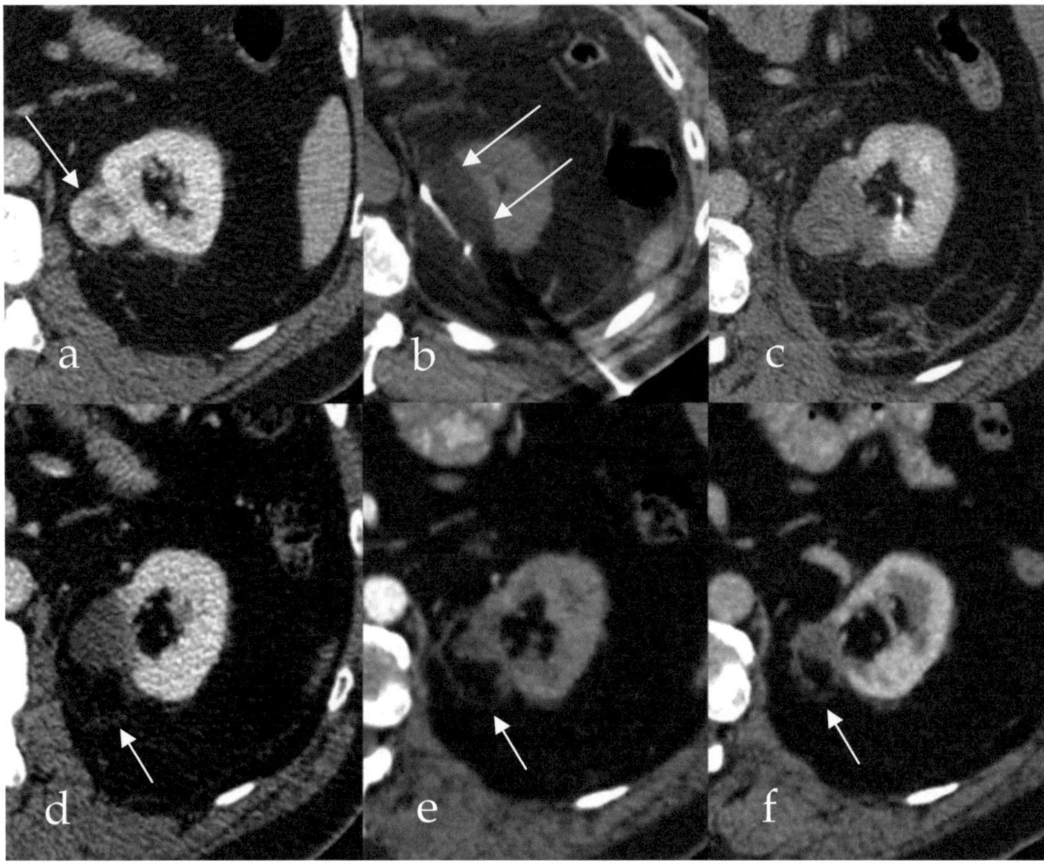

Fig. 1. (a) 62-year-old patient with an incidentally discovered left renal cortical mass (arrow). Separate session biopsy showed conventional clear cell renal cancer. (b) Cryoablation was performed in prone position. This picture is rotated to simulate supine position for ease of comparison. The edge of ice ball is clearly visible in renal parenchyma (white arrows). (c) Contrast enhanced CT image one day after ablation shows lack of enhancement in the ablation zone which covers tumor and an intended margin of renal parenchyma. Follow up contrast enhanced CT images at 3 months (d), 15 months (e) and 30 months after ablation (f). The tumor and adjacent ablated renal parenchyma continuously get smaller in size. A halo at the edge of ablation zone (white arrows) is visible.

MRI is the least commonly used imaging modality for percutaneous ablation. It provides excellent soft tissue resolution with multi planar imaging capability (figure 2). Lack of ionizing radiation is a safety advantage of MRI. MR fluoroscopic sequences can be used for real-time targeting of tumor. MR thermometry can assess cytotoxic tissue temperatures noninvasively. Image-guided percutaneous ablation can be performed using a dedicated interventional magnet, a conventional solenoid magnet, or an open magnet. The ice ball is visualized as a zone of decreased signal intensity on T1- and T2-weighted images. MRI-compatible ablation equipment is available to perform both RFA and cryoablation under MRI guidance (Boss et al., 2005; Miki et al., 2006).

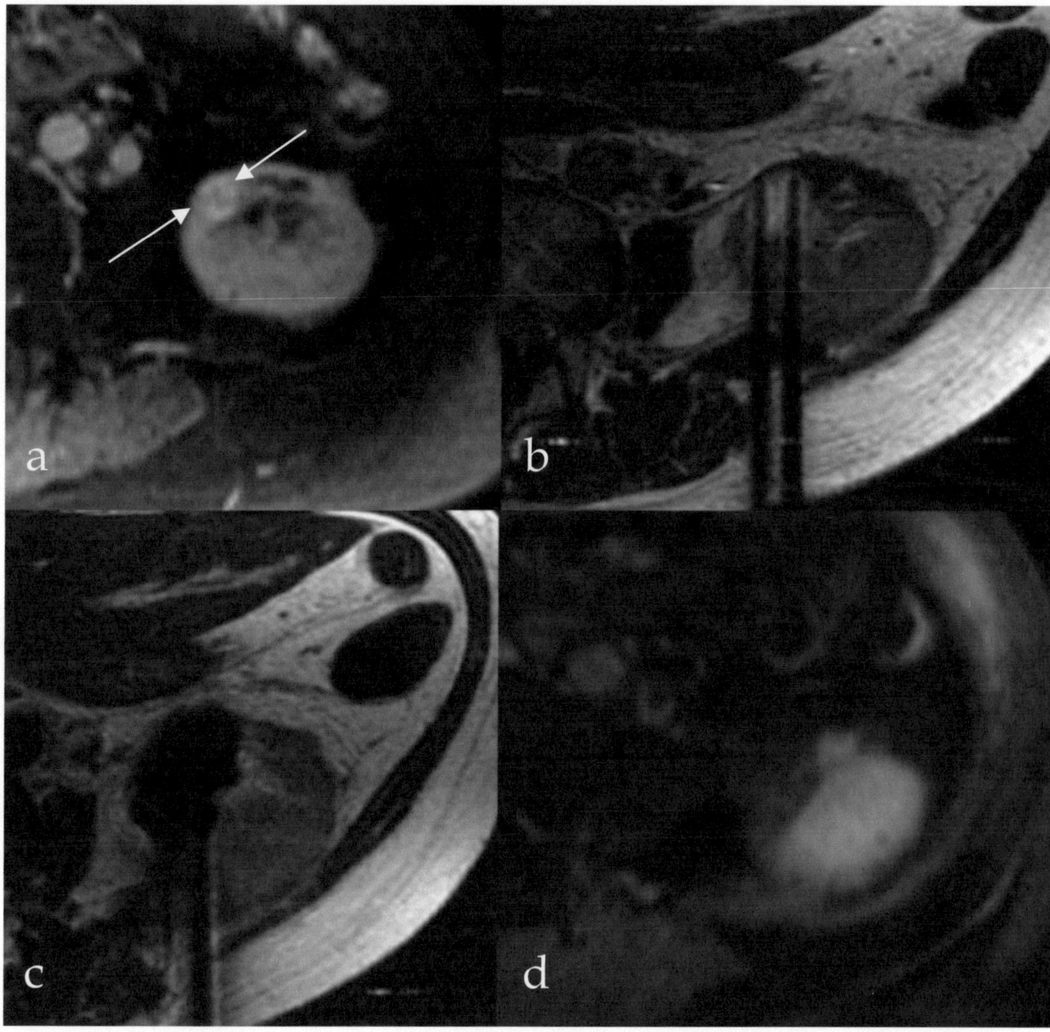

Fig. 2. 77-year-old patient with renal cell cancer of the left kidney (arrows). (a) Contrast enhanced T1 weighted MR scan demonstrates an enhancing tumor in the lower pole of the left kidney. Biopsy confirmed renal cell carcinoma. (b) Two cryoprobes are placed in the tumor under T2 weighted MR guidance. (c) During cryoablation, a low signal "ice ball" encompasses the lesion. Images c and d are rotated to simulate supine position for ease of comparison. (d) Contrast enhanced T1 weighted MRI 3 months after cryoablation demonstrates non-enhancement of the tumor and ablation zone, and shrinkage of the residual mass.

5. Indications and patient selection

Image-guided percutaneous ablations are especially ideal in patients who do not want to undergo surgery, elderly patients with significant medical co-morbidities that preclude them from surgery, patients with renal insufficiency, solitary kidney, transplanted kidney, and multi- focal tumors or patients with diseases such as von Hippel Lindau, which predisposes them to develop multiple renal tumors. Documentation of renal cell carcinoma by needle biopsy is mandatory, as up to 25% of renal masses smaller than 3 cm are benign (American Cancer Society, 2008). Ideally, biopsy should be performed in a session separate from ablation. Tumors should be isolated to kidney with no evidence of vascular invasion or metastases. The best results are anticipated from tumors smaller than 4 cm in diameter, although larger tumors have been successfully ablated. The decision to perform percutaneous ablation is best made as a cooperative multidisciplinary agreement between an interventional radiologist and a urologist.

5.1 Pre procedural evaluation

Before the procedure, a physical exam should be performed, and the patient's medical history should be reviewed. Informed consent is required, and patients must understand that percutaneous ablations are relatively new procedures. Patients are informed about the possibility of retreatment and follow up imaging studies. Allergies to contrast media, antibiotic medications, or anesthetic drugs should also be noted. Laboratory blood tests should include hematocrit, platelet count, prothrombin time, and international normalized ratio (INR), partial thromboplastin time (PTT), and creatinine with calculation of an estimated glomerular filtration rate (eGFR). A platelet count of more than 100,000 per mL, INR of less than 1.5, and normal PTT would ideally be met prior to the procedure. Patients should not be acutely coagulopathic.

Warfarin, aspirin, and clopidogrel should ideally be stopped at least 7 days before the procedure. The operating physician should consult the referring physician prior to withholding anticoagulation medication. In patients with strict warfarin requirements, special arrangements can be made so that ablation is performed using a "heparin window," in which warfarin is held and patients are systemically anticoagulated with heparin until the time of procedure. Patients are instructed to abstain from eating for 6 hours prior to ablation so they are able to receive intravenous moderate sedation or general anesthesia. They may take other routine oral medications with small sips of water. Modification of the insulin regimen in diabetics should be considered during the food restriction period prior to the procedure. Nephrology consultation may be needed prior to ablation in patients with chronic renal insufficiency (estimated GFR less than 60 mL/min).

6. Ablation procedure

The patient should be placed in a comfortable position (prone, supine, lateral decubitus, or with slight elevation of one side) that also facilitates the procedure. Intravenous midazolam and fentanyl are the most commonly used medications for moderate sedation. The drug dosage is titrated for patient comfort and is monitored with telemetry and pulse oximetry by a sedation nurse or anesthesia team. Alternatively and based on institutional policies, percutaneous ablations may be performed under general anesthesia with endotracheal intubation. If desired, a biopsy of the lesion can be performed in the same session prior to the ablation. A challenge with same day biopsy is that bleeding associated with the biopsy may obscure the tumor and potentially affect outcome.

The procedure plan should be outlined by the operating physician before the procedure. The number of probes used for a particular tumor depends on the equipment used and the size of tumor. Placement of more than one probe is often required to cover the entire tumor and the desired rim of surrounding parenchyma. The length of devices extending outside of the patient and their connecting cords, as well as patient positioning and the angle of probe placement, all have major practical implications and should all be planned in advance. Frequently, the injection of intravenous contrast medium during the procedure can help visualize relatively inconspicuous lesions. Smaller doses of iodinated contrast (50 mL) are usually sufficient for CT visualization and can allow for a repeat bolus later in the procedure if necessary. Similarly, there are circumstances when sonographic or MRI contrast agents may be useful.

Adjacent critical structures may be damaged when they are located within the target region. Occasionally, a second percutaneous needle can be inserted and carbon dioxide, water, air, or balloons may be placed to separate bowel, for instance, from the target tumor (Farrell et al., 2003; Kam et al., 2004; Gervais et al., 2005b). It is important not to use saline for hydro dissection in RFA cases, as saline conducts current and may damage organs. Nonionic 5% dextrose in water should be used instead. Certain patient positioning maneuvers or the operating physician's hands may also be used to move away bowel loops from the tumor. Retrograde ureteral stents can be used to circulate warm or cold fluid during the ablation period to provide some protection to the ureter (Cantwell at al., 2008). The probe can also be used as a lever to move the kidney away from adjacent structures (Park & Kim, 2008). If a transpleural approach is inevitable, it can be pursued and any pneumothorax that develops may be treated accordingly. Alternatively, an iatrogenic pneumothorax or hydrothorax can be created to avoid potential damage to the lung.

Unless a tined RFA probe is used, most probes have no tines and produce an oval zone of ablation. After adequate positioning of the probe(s) is complete, the tumor is ablated once or more according to the suggested manufacturer protocol. If the patient's renal function allows, a contrast-enhanced CT or MRI scan may be performed after removing all probes. This will allow for an immediate assessment of the adequacy of the ablation. MRI-guided ablations can also be immediately assessed by MR thermometry. Certain areas with suboptimal ablation can then be immediately re-treated during the same session. At a minimum, it is usually helpful to do a noncontrast scan of the treatment area following removal of probes to assess for complications.

An advantage of cryoablation over heat-based ablation modalities is its relative painlessness (Allaf et al., 2005). This may be of importance for patients who cannot undergo general anesthesia or receive deep moderate sedation due to medical co morbidities.

In contrast to heat-based ablation modalities, the ice ball can be clearly seen with CT (Littrup et al., 2007; Solomon et al., 2004), MRI (Silverman et al., 2005), and ultrasound imaging (Gill et al., 2000). This imaging characteristic allows the operator to ascertain coverage of the tumor more confidently and also to better protect certain nearby critical structures. Because of this feature, cryo ablated lesions tend to have less residual tumor (Marin et al., 2006).

Intravenous contrast is not necessarily needed immediately following cryoablation to verify proper coverage of tumor by the ablation zone. This is a significant advantage for patients with renal insufficiency. The outer edge of the ice ball that is visualized is not cytotoxic. The cytotoxic part of an ice-ball is contained a few millimeters inside the visible edge.

Unlike the heat-based ablation modalities, freezing does not cauterize or coagulate vessels within the ablation zone. Hence, patients may be at slightly higher risk of bleeding during or immediately following cryoablation. For this reason, patients with borderline coagulation status should have laboratory abnormalities more vigorously corrected. One relative limitation of current cryoablation probes is the size of the ablation zone created by a single probe as compared with the same size RFA probe. In general, each 2 mm probe creates an approximately 2 cm diameter of necrosis (Permpongkosol et al., 2007). For this reason, insertion of multiple simultaneous probes is commonly needed to cover the entire tumor and desired margin of surrounding parenchyma. A simple rule-of-thumb is to position the probes about 1 cm from the margin of the tumor and 1 to 2 cm apart from each other, giving priority to the periphery of the tumor (Solomon et al., 2004). It is important to remember that all available cryoablation probes currently have an extension cord attached to them. This cord contains tubing for gases, and in certain versions, temperature sensor wiring as well. The weight of the cord produces torque during and after placement of the probe. When planning for cryoablation, it is important to make sure the trajectory of each probe has enough purchase inside the patient so they are not constantly pulled or deviated by the torque produced by the cord. When positioning the patient for the procedure, it is critical to remember to provide enough space between the patient and gantry so that the equipment does not contact the gantry during the procedure. Additionally, the operating physician will have far more freedom to make fine adjustments during the procedure without having to take the patient out of the gantry repeatedly.

7. Treatment outcomes

Technical success rates of 97 to 100 percent are reported with RFA and cryoablation (Atwell et al., 2008; Boss et al., 2005; Gervais et al., 2005a). In a series of 616 patients, the incidence of residual or recurrent tumor was 13.4 percent with a single radiofrequency ablation and 3.9 percent with a single cryoablation (Gervais et al., 2000). In this series, the overall incidence of residual or recurrent tumor after repeated ablation therapy in all patients was 4.2 percent (Gervais et al., 2000). The overall 2-year survival rate was 82.5 percent, including patients who died of unrelated causes, and the metastasis-free survival rate was 97 percent at 2 years (Gervais et al., 2000). Five-year local and distant tumor-free rate after RFA has been reported at 94 percent (McDougal et al., 2005). Similar success rates are reported with cryoablation, but the mean follow-up time period is shorter at 1 to 2 years (Littrup et al., 2007).

8. Complications

The rate of major complications from percutaneous ablation of renal tumors is about 2 to 6 percent (Atwell et al., 2008; Boss et al., 2005; Johnson at al., 2004). Complications include hemorrhage, pneumothorax, and bowel and nerve injury. In contrast to other heat-based ablation modalities, cryoablation does not cauterize blood vessels within the ablation zone. Therefore, hemorrhage at the ablation zone after removal of probes appears to be slightly more common when compared with heat-based ablation modalities. Hemorrhage after cryoablation is most often self-limited and responds to conservative management. Damage to the renal collecting system and the neighboring structures such as nerves and bowel are among other reported complications.

9. Patient follow up

If the patient's renal function allows, the ablated tumor should be evaluated by CT or MRI without and with intravenous contrast at 1, 3, 6, 12, 18, and 24 months after ablation. Early post ablation studies show the ablation zone as a non-enhancing area surrounded by a thin smooth rim of enhancement (Smith & Gillams; 2008). This rim is considered a physiologic response to thermal ablation and disappears within 3 months (Merkle et al., 2005). Ideally, the ablation zone should include the entire tumor and the expected 5 to 10 mm noncancerous rim; (figure 1 **c**, **d**; figure 2 **d**). The ablation zone appears T1 hyper intense and T2 hypo intense (Uppot et al., 2009; Kawamoto et al, 2009). The ablation zone continues to decrease in size over time (Merkle et al., 2005) (figure 1 **d, e, f**). Complete disappearance of cryoablated tumors over time has been reported (Gill et al., 2005). A thin curvilinear hyper attenuating rim or halo on CT imaging, which is hypo intense on T1-weighted images, is commonly seen parallel to the tumor extending to the perinephric fat (figure 1 **d, e, f**). This halo may persist for several months after treatment (Uppot et al., 2009; Kawamoto et al, 2009). Nodular or irregular enhancement within the ablation zone and enlargement of ablation zone is considered suspicious for residual tumor or recurrence (Kawamoto et al, 2009). These areas may be biopsied and if positive for malignancy they can be treated by ablation.

10. Conclusion

Image-guided percutaneous ablation is a viable option for patients who cannot undergo surgery because of medical co morbidities. Experience with these ablation modalities is promising.

11. References

Allaf ME, Varkarakis IM, Bhayani SB, et al. Pain control requirements for percutaneous ablation of renal tumors: cryoablation versus radiofrequency ablation - initial observations. Radiology 2005;237:366-370

American Cancer Society. Cancer Statistics 2008. Atlanta, GA: American Cancer Society; 2008

Atwell TD, Farrell MA, Leibovich BC, et al. Percutaneous renal cryoablation: experience treating 115 tumors. J Urol 2008;179:2136-2141

Boss A, Clasen S, Kuczyk M, et al. Magnetic resonance guided percutaneous radiofrequency ablation of renal cell carcinomas: a pilot clinical study. Invest Radiol 2005;40: 583-590

Breda A, Finelli A, Janetschek G, Porpiglia F, Montorsi F. Complications of laparoscopic surgery for renal m asses: prevention, management, and comparison with the open experience. Eur Urol 2009;55:836-850

Cantwell CP, Wah TM, Gervais DA, et al. Protecting the ureter during radiofrequency ablation of renal cell cancer: a pilot study of retrograde pyeloperfusion with cooled dextrose 5% in water. J Vase Interv Radiol 2008;19:1034-1040

Chow WH, Devesa SS, Warren JL, Fraumeni JF Jr. Rising incidence of renal cell cancer in the United States. JAMA 1999;281:1628-1631

Deodhar A, Monette S, Single GW Jr, Hamilton WC Jr, Thornton R, Maybody M, Coleman JA, Solomon SB. Renal tissue ablation with irreversible electroporation: preliminary results in a porcine model. Urology. 2011 Mar;77(3):754-60.

Dick EA, Joarder R, DeJode MG, Wragg P, Vale JA, Gedroyc WM. Magnetic resonance imaging-guided laser thermal ablation of renal tumours. BJU Int 2002;90(9):814-822

Farrell MA, Charboneau JW, Callstrom MR, et al. Paranephric water instillation: a technique to prevent bowel injury during percutaneous renal radiofrequency ablation. AJR Am J Roentgenol 2003;181:1315-1317

Fergany AF, Hafez KS, Novick AC. Long-term results of nephron sparing surgery for localized renal cell carcinoma: 10-year follow up. J Urol 2000;163:442-445

Gervais DA, McGovern FJ, Wood BJ, et al. Radiofrequency ablation of renal cell carcinoma: early clinical experience. Radiology 2000;217:665-672

Gervais DA, McGovern FJ, Arellano RS, McDougal WS, Mueller PR. Radiofrequency ablation of renal cell carcinoma. Part 1. Indications, results, and role in patient management over a 6-year period and ablation of 100 tumors. AJR Am J Roentgenol 2005;185:64-71 (a)

Gervais DA, Arellano RS, McGovern FJ, McDougal WS, Mueller PR. Radiofrequency ablation of renal cell carcinoma: part 2, lessons learned with ablation of 100 tumors. AJR Am J Roentgenol 2005;185:72-80 (b)

Gill IS, Novick AC, Meraney AM, et al. Laparoscopic renal cryoablation in 32 patients. Urology 2000;56:748-753

Gill IS, Remer EM, Hasan WA, et al. Renal cryoablation: outcome at 3 years. J Urol 2005;173:1903-1907

Gill IS, Kavoussi LR, Lane BR, et al. Comparison of 1,800 laparoscopic and open partial nephrectomies for single renal tumors. J Urol 2007;178:41-46

Gontero P, Joniau S, Zitella A, Tailly T, Tizzani A, Van Poppel H, Kirkali Z. Ablative therapies in the treatment of small renal tumors : how far from standard of care ? Urol Oncol 2010; 28: 251-259

Hui GC, Tuncali K, Tatli S, Morrison PR, Silverman SG. Comparison of percutaneous and surgical approaches to renal tumor ablation: metaanalysis of effectiveness and complication rates. J Vase Interv Radiol 2008;19:1311-1320

Janzen NK, Kim HL, Figlin RA, et al. Surveillance after radical or nephron sparing surgery for localized renal cell carcinoma and management of recurrent disease. Urol Clin North Am 2003;30:843-852

Janzen NK, Perry KT, Han KR, et al. The effects of intentional cryoablation and radiofrequency ablation of renal tissue involving the collecting system in a porcine model. J Urol 2005;173:1368-1374

Johnson DB, Solomon SB, Su LM, et al. Defining the complications of cryoablation and radiofrequency ablation of small renal tumors: a multi-institutional review. J Urol 2004; 172:874-877

Joniau S, Tailly T, Goeman L, Blyweert W, Gontero P, Joyce A. Kidney radiofrequency ablation for small renal tumors: oncologic efficacy. J. Endourol. 2010; 24: 721-728.

Kam AW, Littru p PJ, Walther MM, et al. Thermal protection during percutaneous thermal abla tion of renal cell carcinoma. J Vase Interv Radiol 2004;15:753-758

Kawamoto S, Solomon SB, Bluemke DA, Fishman EK. Computed tomography and magnetic resonance imaging appearance of renal neoplasms after radiofrequency ablation and cryoablation. Semin Ultrasound CT MR 2009;30:67-77

Klatte T, Marberger M. High-intensity focused ultrasound for the treatment of renal masses: current status and future potential. Curr Opin Urol 2009;19:188-191

Littrup PJ, Ahmed A, Aoun HD, et al. CT-guided percutaneous cryotherapy of renal masses. J Vasc Interv Radiol 2007;18:383-392

Luciani LG, Cestari R, Tallarigo C. Incidental renal cell carcinoma-age and stage characterization and clinical implications: study of 1092 patients (1982-1997). Urology 2000;56:58-62

Marberger M, Schatzl G, Kranston D, Kennedy JE. Extracorporeal ablation of renal tumors with high intensity focused ultrasound. BJU Int 2005;95:52-55

Marin SF, Ahrar K, Cadeddu JA, et al. Residual and recurrent disease following renal energy ablative therapy: a multi-institutional study. J Urol 2006;176:1973-1977

Maybody M, Solomon SB. Image-guided percutaneous cryoablation of renal tumors. Tech Vasc Interv Radiol. 2007;10:140-148

McDougal WS, Gervais DA, McGovern FJ, Mueller PR. Long-term follow-up of patients with renal cell carcinoma treated with radio frequency ablation with curative intent. J Urol 2005;174:61-63

Merkle EM, Nour SG, Lewin JS. MR imaging follow-up after percutaneous radiofrequency ablation of renal cell carcinoma: findings in 18 patients during first 6 months. Radiology 2005;235:1065-1071

Miki K, Shimomura T, Yamada H, et al. Percutaneous cryoablation of renal cell carcinoma guided by horizontal open magnetic resonance imaging. Int J Urol 2006;13:880-884

Mouraviev V, Joniau S, Van Poppel H, Polascik TJ. Current status of minimally invasive ablative techniques in the treatment of small renal tumors. Eur Urol 2007; 51: 328-336

Pantuck AJ, Zisman A, Belldegrun AS. The changing natural history of renal cell carcinoma. J Urol 2001;166:1611-1623

Park BK, Kim CK. Using an electrode as a lever to increase the distance between renal cell carcinoma and bowel during CT-guided radiofrequency ablation. Eur Radiol 2008;18: 743-746

Permpongkosol S, Nicol TL, Link RE, et al. Differences in ablation size in porcine kidney, liver, and lung after cryoablation using the same ablation protocol. AJ R Am J Roentgenol 2007;188:1028-1032

Rubinsky B, Onik G, Mikus P. Irreversible electroporation: a new ablation modality: clinical implications. Technol Cancer Res Treat 2007;6:37-48

Silverman SG, Tuncali K, van Sonnenberg E, et al. Renal tumors MR imaging-guided percutaneous cryotherapy - initial experience in 23 patients. Radiology 2005;236: 716-724

Simon CJ, Dupuy DE, Mayo-Smith WW. Microwave ablation: principles and applications. Radiographics 2005;25: S69-S83

Smith S, Gillams A. Imaging appearances following thermal ablation. Clin Radiol 2008;63:1-11

Solomon SB, Chan DY, Jarrett TW. Percutaneous cryotherapy of kidney tumors. Am J Urol Rev 2004;2:369-371

Spaliviero M, Moinzadeh A, Gill IS. Laparoscopic cryotherapy for renal tumors. Technol Cancer Res Treat 2004; 3:177-180

Uppot RN, Silverman SG, Zagoria RJ, Tuncali K, Childs DD, Gervais DA. Imaging-guided percutaneous ablation of renal cell carcinoma: a primer of how we do it. AJR Am J Roentgenol 2009;192:1558-1570

6

Radiofrequency Ablation for Renal Tumor, Past, Present and Future

Vilar D. Gallego
Hospital General Castellon
Spain

1. Introduction

Cancer of the kidney is the third most common cancer of the urinary tract and accounts for 3.5% of all malignancies. With an estimated 51,190 new cases occurring in 2007 and 12,890 deaths attributable to the disease, renal cell carcinoma (RCC) is the most lethal of all genitourinary tumors (1).

The clinical diagnosis of RCC is radiographic, and effective imaging of the kidneys can be achieved by ultrasound, computed tomography (CT), or magnetic resonance imaging (MRI) (2). Because of the increased use of diagnostic imaging for the evaluation of patients with abdominal symptoms, incidentally discovered small renal masses (SMRs) are being diagnosed with greater frequency (3) and may account for up to 66% of RCC diagnoses (4). Thus, an increased incidence of RCC over the last 30 years has been associated with stage migration and a concurrent rise in rates of surgical intervention (5). Unfortunately, despite earlier diagnosis and treatment, cancer-specific survival (CSS) and overall survival have not improved significantly, this could be due to the fact that we deliver less treatmentfor solid kidney tumorsthan in the past (6).

Surgical resection remains the standard of care for clinically localized RCC because of the favorable prognosis associated with surgery and the relative ineffectiveness of systemic therapy. Patients who undergo radical or partial nephrectomy for SRMs (tumors classified as pathologic T1a [pT1a], tumors 4 cm) exhibit 5-year CSS rates in excess of 95%. Laparoscopic approaches to partial nephrectomy have produced similarly favorable early results (7).

Recently, minimally invasive ablative technologies have emerged as potential treatment options for clinically localized RCC. The question of whether in situ ablative technologies (8) can replace excision for the treatment of small renal tumours remains unanswered. The reported advantages of ablative approaches over extirpative techniques include reduction of perioperative morbidity, shorter hospital stay and faster recovery time. The main advantage of ablative techniques, however, would be to offer treatment to patients who are otherwise not candidates for invasive extirpative techniques. Radiofrequency ablation (RFA) is a minimally invasive treatment for localized cancer in which a small needle attached to a device that delivers radiofrequency energy is inserted into a tumour to destroy the cancerous tissue while the patient is sedated or under general anesthesia. The procedure is usually performed percutaneously with image guidance using computed tomography (CT)

or ultrasonography (9). Although these newer nephron-sparing techniques appear to be promising, the majority of published studies are single-institution series with relatively few numbers of patients.
Although treatment options for low-stage RCC have expanded in recent years, their proper application and their affect on the biology of SRMs has yet to be defined fully. Here we analyze the combined published data regarding RFA as treatment of SRMs.

2. History of RFA

Minimally invasive tumor ablation therapy for focal malignancies encompasses several specific objectives. Most importantly, through the application of energy or chemicals, the primary goal of most ablation procedures is to eradicate all viable malignant cells within a designated target volume. As such, one substantial advantage of percutaneous ablative therapies over conventional surgical resection is the potential to remove or destroy only a minimal amount of normal tissue. This is also useful when nephron-sparing treatments are needed in patients with von Hippel–Lindau syndrome, who are prone to the development of multiple renal cell carcinomas and in patients with primary lung malignancies in the setting of extensive underlying emphysema and limited lung function.Currently Indications for minimally invasive techniques, including RFA, are: small, incidentally found, renal cortical lesions in elderly patients; patients with a genetic predisposition for developing multiple tumours; patients with bilateral tumours; patients with a solitary kidney at high risk of complete loss of renal function following surgical tumour resection (LE: 2b). Contraindications to the above-mentioned procedures include: poor life expectancy of < 1 year; multiple metastases; low possibility of successful treatment due to size or location of tumour. In general, tumours > 3 cm or tumours in the hilum, near the proximal ureter or the central collecting system are not typically recommended for ablative techniques via a percutaneous approach. (10). RFA of an exophytic renal mass before open radical nephrectomy was described first in 1997 (11) and the first report of RFA as sole treatment for a renal tumor was published in 1999 (12). Although RFA has been applied using open, laparoscopic, or percutaneous approaches under ultrasound, CT, or MRI guidance, the current literature describes percutaneous access in approximately 94% of patients who underwent renal RFA.

3. RFA electrodes and generators

Three types of RF electrodes are currently available commercially: two brands of retractable needle electrodes (model 70 and model 90 Starburst XL needles, RITA Medical Systems, Mountain View, CA, USA; LeVeen needle electrode, Boston Scientific, Boston, MA, USA) and an internally cooled electrode (Cool-Tip RF electrode; Radionics, Burlington, MA, USA) (13).
The needle electrodes of RITA consist of a 14-gauge insulated outer needle that houses nine retractable curved electrodes of various lengths. When the electrodes are extended, the device assumes the approximate configuration of a Christmas tree. Nine of the electrodes are hollow and contain thermocouples in their tips in order to measure the temperature of adjacent tissue. The alternating electric current generator comes in a 250-W model at 460 kHz (Model 1500X RF Generator, RITA Medical Systems). The ablation algorithm is based on temperature at the tips of the electrodes. After the ablation cycle is completed, a

temperature reading from the extended electrodes in excess of 50°C at 1 min is considered to indicate satisfactory ablation.

Another RFA device (LeVeen Needle Electrode; Radiotherapeutics. OWL universal RF System URP-3AP: figure I) has retractable curved electrodes and an insulated 17-gauge outer needle that houses 10 solid retractable curved electrodes that, when deployed, assume the configuration of an umbrella. The electrodes are manufactured in different lengths (2- to 4.0-cm umbrella diameter). The alternating electric current generator is 200 W operated at 480 kHz (RF 3000; Boston Scientific). The ablation algorithm is based on tissue impedance, and ablation is considered successful if the device impedes out.

The third RFA device (Cool-Tip radiofrequency electrode; Radionics) has an insulated hollow 17-gauge needle with an exposed needle tip of variable length (2- or 3-cm). The tip of the needle contains a thermocouple to record the temperature of adjacent tissue. The shaft of the needle has two internal channels to allow the needle to be perfused with chilled water. In an attempt to further increase the size of the ablation area, the manufacturer placed three of the cooled needles in a parallel triangular cluster with a common hub. The generator has a peak power output of 200 W and is operated at 480 kHz (CC-1; Radionics). The ablation algorithm is based on tissue impedance, and ablation is considered successful if the device impedes out. As a result, successful ablations usually increase the temperature of the ablated tissue to above 60°C.

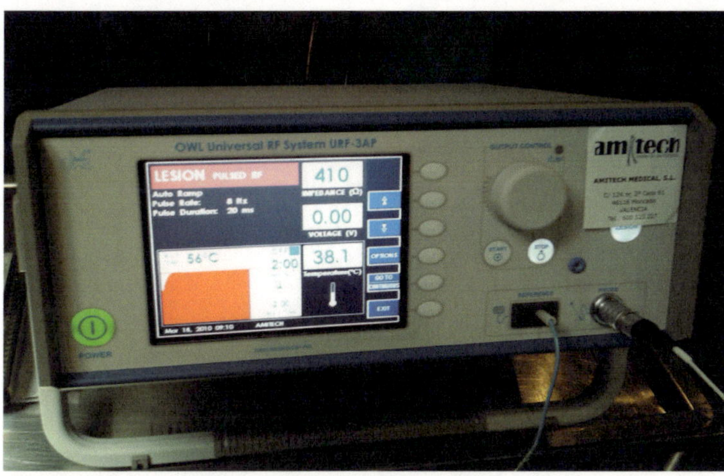

Fig. 1. RF generator: OWL universal RF System URP-3AP

4. Mechanism of action

Radiofrequency (RF) energy can be used to rapidly create highly localized lesions via a temperature-based or an impedance-based system. Both systems rely on the creation of a closed electrical circuit. The cytotoxic mechanism in both involves desiccation due to high intracellular temperatures. High-frequency current flows from a needle electrode to the surrounding tissue, resulting in ionic agitation, which leads to accelerated molecular friction, which producesheat. Heat induces immediate cellular damage, leading to coagulative necrosis. Energy returns to the RF generator via a return pad that com- pletes the circuit.

The macroscopic and microscopic findings following RF treatment correlate (14). Macroscopically, after RF treatment, kidneys demonstrate a gray-white area of necrosis surrounding a central cavity containing both areas of hemorrhage and necrotic debris.
Clear demarcation exists between the induced lesion and the surrounding normal parenchyma. Shortly after RF ablation, intense stromal and epithelial edema with marked hypereosinophilia and pyknosis are present, accompanied by microvascular thrombosis and coag- ulative necrosis. Chronic lesions demonstrate dense fibrosis.

5. Technique

Monopolar needles are coupled with secondary hooks to create spherical lesions (Figure II-III). An insulating shaft protects normal tissue. Tissue temperature measurements are made via thermo-couples located at the tip of the needles. Electrode temperatures at approximately 100°C are generally required in order to assure temperatures of at least 60°C at the periphery of the ablated lesion (15). Multiprobe, hooked, and bipolar arrays; intraparenchymal saline injection; and internally cooled electrodes have all been developed to increase the size of the lesion created. Polascik and colleagues (16) introduced the modified technique of saline perfusion of tissue during RFA.

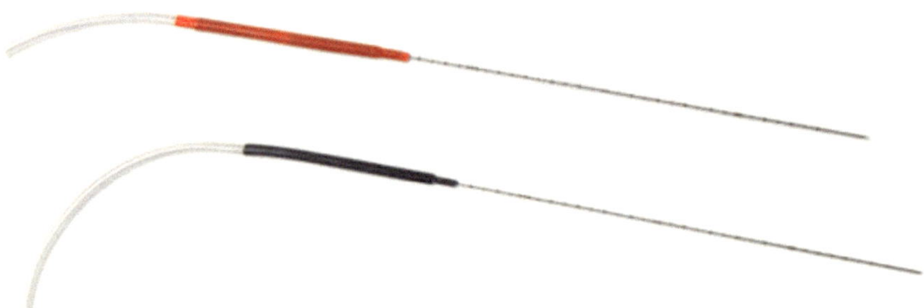

Fig. 2. Monopolar needles

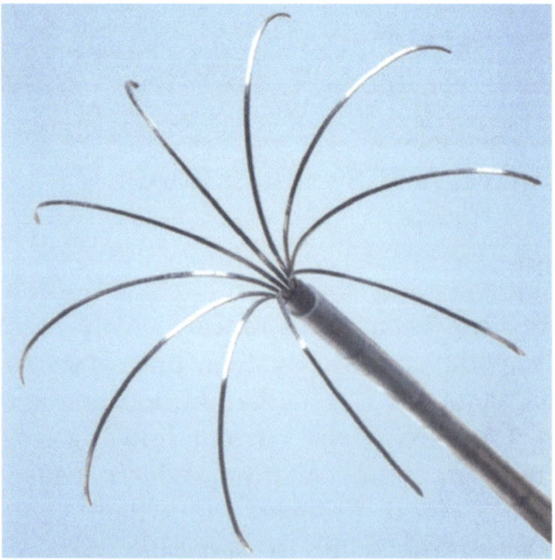

Fig. 3. Monopolar needles

5.1 Electrodes

Most RF ablation systems today operate in a monopolar mode by using two different types of electrodes: interstitial electrodes (hereafter, electrode) and dispersive electrodes on the skin surface (also known as ground pads). The electrode delivers energy to the tumor, creating a volume of high current density and localized heating.

Monopolar electrode designs include both straight insulated needles with an exposed metallic tip and multitined electrodes. Internally cooled electrodes use a single needle, in which fluid is circulated inside the electrode's active tip, and temperatures at the electrode-tissue interface are reduced. Internally cooled needles are now used by the Cool-tip system (Valleylab by Covidien, Boulder, Colo).

In contrast, electrodes with multiple tines emanating from a single electrode sheath or handle assembly aim to distribute energy spatially (17).

Crowley and colleagues (18) showed minimal morbidity and allowed monitoring and control of ablation with impedance-based system in a porcine model.

The ability to monitor the lesioning process during RFA using real-time ultrasound is debatable. Some authors (19) reported that in a saline-infused RFA, a bubbling effect in the area of the treatment may be ultra-sonographically imaged as an area of increased echogenicity. Ultrasound is not useful for intraoperative monitoring. Posttreatment lesions appeared as a distinct hyperechoic zone, an area of bright echogenic foci, or a heterogeneous area of mild hyperechogenicity.

6. What about clinical outcomes?

6.1 Predictive factors for success of RFA

Tumor size is an important predictor of successful treatment in RF ablation of renal tumors. Despite advances in electrode design, the successful ablation of tumors, greater than 4 cm in diameter, has been a challenge (20). Therefore, smaller renal tumors are ideal candidates for an RF ablation. On the other hand, the larger tumors require multiple overlapping ablations and, in some cases, return visits for additional ablation sessions (20).

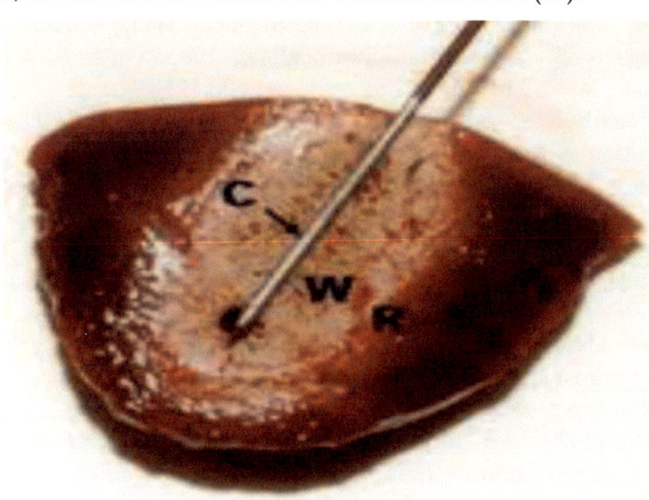

Fig. 4. "Owen effect": "R": red zone=kidney; "C": center of the lession; "W":white zone=fibrotic capsula

The location of the tumor within the kidney may also play an important role in the efficacy of the RF ablation treatment for renal masses, and may influence the success of an ablation. A central tumor ablation fails more frequently because of a heat sink effect, in which a regional vascular flow reduces the extent of the thermally induced coagulation (21). By contrast, exophytic lesions are surrounded by perirenal fat, which serves as a heat insulator and allows the achievement of higher temperatures during RF ablation. This phenomenon was first described in liver tumors and referred to as the "owen effect" (Figure IV) where hepatic tumors surrounded by a fibrotic capsule and surrounding cirrhotic liver tissue are more easily treated (22). As a result of this phenomenon, exophytic renal tumors have an increased likelihood of successful ablation. Therefore, size and location are good predictors of success, with small exophytic renal tumors being the most suitable candidates for RF ablation (23).

6.2 Clinical outcomes

Stern et al. (24) published their results in 37 ASA 1-2 patients. Only one patient had a local recurrence in a period over 2 years and he was treated by radical nephrectomy without recurrence after 1 year follow- up. The same author compared intermediate-term results of partial nephrectomy and radiofrequency ablation and concluded that 3-year oncological outcomes were similar (25).

Gervais and colleagues (26) published a series of 85 patients with the treatment of 100 tumors percutaneously. One local recurrence was seen. Indeed, 100% of the tumors smaller than 3 cm achieved complete ablation while only 25% of tumors greater than 5 cm were completely treated. Another paper of the same group, a cohort of 16 patients was reported with the longest term follow-up available (4.6 years). Five patients died of unrelated causes and the 5-year cáncer specific survival was 100%. Zagoria et al. (27) obtained complete ablation (absence of contrast enhancement in the tumors on CT or MRI) in 96% of tumors altough residual tumors were observed in 30% of those larger than 3.7 cm in a follow-up of 13.8 months.

Lucas et al (28) found a 6.97% of local recurrence and it was higher than in Bensalah´s serie (29) with a global rate of 2.63% of local recurrence, Weight et al (30) described a radiographic success in 85% and no mailgnant cells on biopsy after RFA in 65% of patients and Breen et al (31) an overall technical success rate of 90.47%.

Traver et al. (32) recently reported outcomes of 73 renal tumours in 65 patients treated with PRFA under CT guidance. Mean tumor size was size 2.9 cm. Although initial tumour control was obtained in 84.9%, 5 of 11 initial treatment failures were successfully retreated, 4 were followed conservatively, 1 required nephrectomy, and 1 patient died of unrelated causes. In patients with initial tumour control, recurrence occurred in 8.1%. Matsumoto et al. (33) got better results in a serie of 109 small renal tumours (91 patients) treated with CT-guided percutaneous . Mean tumour size was 2.4. The initial ablation was successful in 98% with two incomplete ablations successfully re-ablated. With at least 1 yr of follow-up, 60% had preoperatively biopsy proven RCC. In this group, one local recurrence was detected during a mean follow-up of 19.4 months and in those with known RCC, none had evidence of distant progression. The local recurrence was successfully re-ablated such that all 109 cases had no clinical or radiographic evidence of disease at last follow-up. Gallego et al. (34) presented a serie of 11 renal tumors in 9 patients. Mean tumor size was higher than in most of the papers reported previously (3.5 cm). In 2 patients two new RF session was needed. 9 tumors with treatment considered effective. Mean follow-up was 17.5 months (3-52 months).

One patient had local recurrence at 14 months and needed a laparoscopic radical nephrectomy and two patients developed lung metastases 41.5 months after RF. There were no clinically relevant complications.

RFA performed intraoperatively immediately before surgical nephrectomy using standard machines and ablation proto- cols did not result in complete cell kill, with persistence of viable tumor cells based on NADH staining varying from 50% to 100% in 2 small series (35). Recently, Klingler et al. (36) found incomplete ablation in 4/17 (14%) renal tumors receiving LRFA before undergoing LPN and concluded that RFA failures can occur also with modern high-energy equipment, thus limiting the indication of this MI thermoablative T to selected high risk patients.

6.3 Follow-up

Radiographic follow-up after RFA is currently the most common means of assessing treatment effect (37). Enhancement on postcontrast imaging is considered evidence of incompletely treated disease. Some centers have performed biopsy after ablation to assess for viable disease, whereas others have relied solely on radiographic evaluation (Figure V)(38). Although the presence of macroscopically viable disease may be detectable on follow-up imaging immediately after ablation, microscopic disease may require a longer duration of surveillance to become apparent. This may explain recent data suggesting that viable tumor may be present on postablation biopsy despite lack of radiographic enhancement. The Working Group on Image-Guided Tumor Ablation has used the term local tumor progression to indicate incomplete tumor destruction regardless of the time it takes for enduring disease to become evident clinically (39). Thus, the ultimate rate of treatment failure after salvage ablation remains to be fully defined. Furthermore, it is likely that ablation techniques have undergone refinement with increased experience; therefore, published series may not truly reflect contemporary results.

When comparing the rates of local disease persistence it is important to consider that nonuniform criteria may have been used to define recurrence after ablation. Although the majority of series used contrast-enhanced imaging to determine treatment effect, the definition of ablative success has been called into question by studies that have demonstrated viable tumor on postablation biopsy despite a lack of enhancement on imaging (40). Perhaps the true rate of local disease progression could be determined more accurately if biopsy were included routinely in postablation surveillance protocols.

The context in which the technical success of renal ablation is evaluated must include consideration of the emerging body of data regarding the observation or active surveillance of SRMs in elderly or infirm populations. Although published series addressing the natural history of small renal tumors under active surveillance report some variability in the clinical behavior of observed SRMs (growth rates of 0.09-0.86 cm per year), a meta-analysis of clinically localized tumors determined an overall median growth rate of 0.28 cm per year for observed lesions across multiple published series (41). Moreover, it has been reported that from 26% to 33% of enhancing renal masses demonstrate zero net growth when observed over a median of 29 months (42). It is note-worthy that only 1% of lesions reported in the active surveillance literature have demonstrated progression to metastatic disease in the absence of treatment. This information raises the possibility of an over-treatment bias for SRMs and suggests that treatment may not have an impact on the biologic potential of many lesions (43), but it is clear that today, with the availability of minimal invasive techniques like percutaneous RFA only in patients who have competing health risks, radiographic **surveillance** may be an acceptable initial approach, and delayed intervention may be reserved for patients who have tumors that exhibit significant linear or volumetric growth. (44)

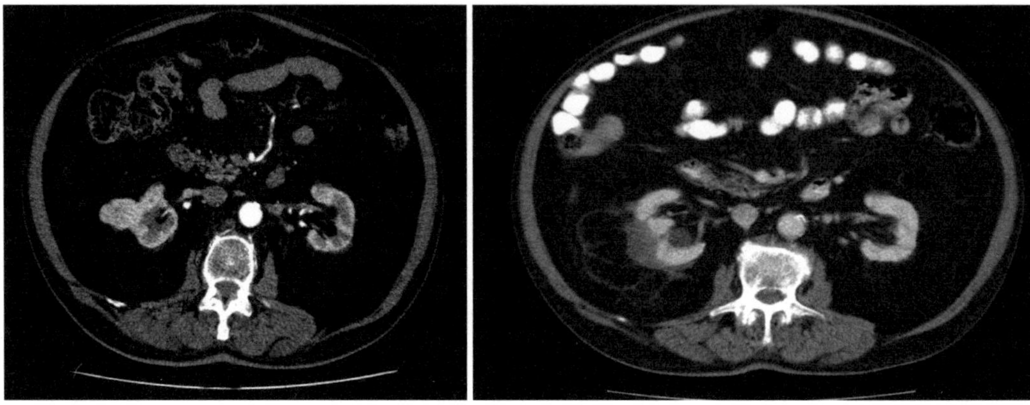

Fig. 5. Renal tumor previous and after RF ablation, after RF there is no contrast enhacement at CT scan

6.4 Effects on renal function

In addition to their minimally invasive nature, another primary benefit of ablative therapy for renal tumors is the potential for preservation of renal func- tion. However, to our knowledge, few studies to date have examined the effects of kidney ablation on re- nal function. Gill et al (45) examined 56 patients with 3- year follow-up after renal cryoablation and reported preoperative and postoperative serum creatinine levels of 1.2 mg/dL and 1.4 mg/dL, respectively. In 10 patients who had solitary kidneys in that series, the mean preoperative and postoperative serum creatinine levels were 2.2 mg/dL and 2.6 mg/dL, respectively, and 13 patients with baseline renal insufficiency demonstrated levels of 3 mg/dL and 2.7 mg/dL, respectively (46). In another series of 14 patients who underwent cryoablation in a solitary kidney, no adverse effect on renal function was noted, although 3 lesions required repeat treatment for incomplete ablation (41). A serie that examined the effects of RFA on 16 patients with a solitary kidney demonstrated a decrease in the mean glomerular filtration rate from 54.2 mL per minute per 1.73 m2 preoperatively to 47.5 mL per minute per 1.73 m2 at last follow-up (47). Similarly, Jacobsohn et al (48) studied 16 patients who underwent RFA in a solitary kidney and demon- strated a 13.3% change in creatinine clearance within 1 week after ablation and a 9.1% change at a mean follow-up of 15.3 months with 1 patient developing chronic renal failure. The ability to spare nephrons maximally remains a careful balance against the possibility of insufficient tumor destruction.

6.5 Complications

Recent data have revealed that two potential serious renal complications associated with RFA are urinoma and a proximal ureteral stricture. Traver et al. (49) reported 2 cases of ureteral strictures from a series of 73 tumours treated with percutaneous RFA: Matsumoto et al. (33) in 1 case of 91, and Weizer et al. (50) in 1 case of 24 patients, respectively. Another major complication that has occurred is colon injury as described by Weizer et al. (50) in 2 of 24 patients undergoing percutaneous RFA. Other minor complications reported are a small perinephric haematoma and pneumothoraces (51).

7. Future

Ablation research has historically focused on creating larger or more uniform zones of ablation that are reproducible in many situations through device and application development, but device engineering is always constrained by the physiology of the target. New approaches to augment device performance by altering the underlying tissue physiology, optimizing energy delivery, or combining ablative therapies with other treatments, such as radiation or drug therapies, to increase ablation size, uniformity, or treatment specificity have been described.

Many recent investigations have centered on altering underlying tumor physiology as a means to advance thermal ablation. Most studies to date have focused on the effects of tissue characteristics in the setting of temperature-based therapies in general, such as tissue perfusion and thermal conductivity, and system-specific characteristics, such as electrical conductivity for RF-based ablation.

7.1 Tissue perfusión

The foremost factor limiting thermal ablation of tumors continues to be tissue blood flow, which acts as a heat sink and reduces the volume of tissue heated to target temperature, either through large blood vessels or capillary-mediated perfusion. Promising antiangiogenic therapies, such as sorafenib, are also starting to be studied as combination therapies with ablation, with similar encouraging results in animals (52).

7.2 Thermal conductivity

Increased thermal conductivity, such as that in cystic lesions, results in fast heat transmission (ie, heat dissipation), with potentially incomplete and heterogeneous tumor heating. Different tumor and organ characteristics may also make a 1-cm ablative margin difficult to achieve (53).

7.3 Electrical conductivity

Altering the electrical environment immediately around the RF electrode with ionic agents can increase electrical conductivity prior to or during RF ablation, allow greater energy deposition, and, therefore, increase coagulation volume (54).

7.4 Combining percutaneous ablation with other therapies

While substantial efforts have been made in modifying ablation systems and the biologic environment to improve the clinical utility of percutaneous ablation, limitations in clinical efficacy persist. For example, with further long-term follow-up of patients undergoing ablation therapy, there has been an increased incidence of detection of progressive local tumor growth for all tumor types and sizes despite initial indications of adequate therapy, suggesting that there are residual foci of viable untreated disease in a substantial number of cases (55). The ability to achieve complete and uniform eradication of all malignant cells remains a key barrier to clinical success, and therefore, strategies that can increase the completeness of tumor destruction with RF ablation, even for small lesions, are needed. Investigators have sought to improve results by combining thermal ablation with adjuvant therapies, such as radiation and chemotherapy (56).

RFA qith chemotherapy: The underlying mechanisms of this synergy are multifactorial. Improved intratumoral drug delivery occurs with use of a liposomal carrier owing to increased circulation time, increased drug release with thermosensitive liposome types, and the well-documented vascular effects of sublethal hyperthermia in the peripheral treatment zone (57). Additionally, the cytotoxic effects of the chemotherapy agent combine with the heat-induced reduction in cellular reparative mechanisms to increase apoptosis (58). Finally, study results suggest that there are independent heat-related cytotoxic effects of the liposome itself (58). This preliminary success with combination therapy may be augmented by the development of new targeting vehicles, including several polymer-based temperature-dependent delivery systems currently under investigation (59).

RFA with radiation therapy: Previous data in the literature have demonstrated increased tumor destruction with external beam radiation therapy and low-temperature hyperthermia (60, 61). Findings in experimental animal studies have demonstrated increased tumor necrosis, reduced tumor growth, and improved animal survival with combined therapy when compared with either therapy alone (62). Preliminary clinical studies in primary lung malignancies confirm the synergistic effects of these therapies. Potential causes for the synergy include the sensitization of the tumor to subsequent radiation owing to the increased oxygenation resulting from hyperthermia-induced increased blood flow to the tumor (63). Future research is needed to identify the optimal temperature for ablation, the optimal radiation dose, and the most effective method of administering radiation therapy (eg, external beam radiation therapy, brachytherapy, or yttrium microspheres) on an organ-by-organ basis.

8. Conclusions

Excision remains the reference standard for the treatment of the small renal mass. Most studies pertaining to probe ablation provide level 3–4 evidence. RFA is a suitable and promising therapy in patients with small renal tumours (< 4 cm) who are considered to be poor candidates for more involved surgery. Long-term data on oncological control is lacking and more rigorous head-to-head trials are needed to determine the exact role of RFA in the treatment algorithm of small renal masses.

Concerns about residual tumour and local recurrences after RFA need to be addressed. As we have seen there are no sistematic follow-up strategies after RFA of renal tumors. Usually, local recurrence and development of metastasis are assessed by images and many definitions of radiographic success is being used. This arbritary method of follow up has been inadequate for determining complete ablation since positive biopsies have been reported. In future, molecular markers will also be considered for this purpose. Ideally, surveillance after ablations as well as reporting of outcomes, technique and histological confirmation should be standarized to make posible as better follow up and comparision of RFA series with surgery.

9. Acknowledgment

To Juan, my father, my mentor, my friend. To Sebastian, to his great diary lessons of how to listen, to quiet, when to talk and how to love, we will never forget you.

10. References

[1] Jemal A, Siegel R, Ward E, Murray T, Xu J, Thun MJ. Cancer statistics, 2007. CA Cancer J Clin. 2007;57:43-66

[2] Chawla SN, Crispen PL, Hanlon AL, Greenberg RE, Chen DY, Uzzo RG. The natural history of observed enhancing renal masses: meta-analysis and review of the world litera- ture. J Urol. 2006;175:425-431.

[3] Jayson M, Sanders H. Increased incidence of serendipi tously discovered renal cell carcinoma. Urology. 1998;51: 203-205.

[4] Volpe A, Panzarella T, Rendon RA, Haider MA, Kondylis FI, Jewett MA. The natural history of incidentally detected small renal masses. Cancer. 2004;100:738-745.

[5] Hollingsworth JM, Miller DC, Daignault S, Hollenbeck BK. Rising incidence of small renal masses: a need to reassess treatment effect. J Natl Cancer Inst. 2006;98:1331-1334.

[6] Hock LM, Lynch J, Balaji KC. Increasing incidence of all stages of kidney cancer in the last 2 decades in the United States: an analysis of surveillance, epidemiology and end results program data. J Urol. 2002 Jan;167(1):57-60.

[7] Lane BR, Gill IS. 7-year oncological outcomes after laparoscopic and open partial nephrectomy. J Urol. 2010 Feb;183(2):473-9

[8] Pavlovich CP, Walther MM, Choyke PL, et al. Percutaneous radio frequency ablation of small renal tumours: initial results. J Urol 2002;167:10-5.

[9] Mahnken AH, Rohde D, Brkovic D, Günther RW, Tacke JA. Percutaneous radiofrequency ablation of renal cell carcinoma: preliminary results. Acta Radiol. 2005 Apr;46(2):208-14.

[10] B. Ljungberg, N. Cowan, D.C. Hanbury, M. Hora, M.A. Kuczyk, A.S. Merseburger, P.F.A. Mulders, J-J. Patard, I.C. Sinescu. Guidelines on Renal Cell Carcinoma. Eur Urol. 2010.

[11] Zlotta AR, Wildschutz T, Raviv G, et al. Radiofrequency in- terstitial tumor ablation (RITA) is a possible new modality for treatment of renal cancer: ex vivo and in vivo experience. J Endourol. 1997;11:251-258.

[12] McGovern FJ, Wood BJ, Goldberg SN, Mueller PR. Radio frequency ablation of renal cell carcinoma via image guided needle electrodes. J Urol. 1999;161:599-600.

[13] McGhana JP, Dodd GD 3rd. Radiofrequency ablation of the liver: current status. AJR Am J Roentgenol. 2001;176:3–16.

[14] Zlotta AR, Djavan B, Matos C, Noel JC, Peny MO, Silverman DE, Marberger M, Schulman CC. Percutaneous transperineal radiofrequency ablation of prostate tumour: safety, feasibility and pathological effects on human prostate cancer. Br J Urol. 1998 Feb;81(2):265-75.

[15] Walther MC, Shawker TH, Libutti SK, et al. A phase 2 study of radio frequency interstitial tis- sue ablation of localized tumors. J Urol. 2000;163:1424–1427.

[16] Polascik TJ, Hamper U, Lee BR, et al. Ablation of renal tumors in a rabbit model with intersti- tial saline-augmented radiofrequency energy: preliminary report of a new technology. Urology. 1999;53:465–472.

[17] Gulesserian T, Mahnken AH, Schernthaner R, et al. Comparison of expandable electrodes in percutaneous radiofrequency ablation of renal cell carcinoma. Eur J Radiol 2006;59(2):133–139.

[18] Crowley JD, Shelton J, Iverson AJ, et al. Laparoscopic and computed tomography-guid- ed percutaneous radiofrequency ablation of renal tissue: acute and chronic effects in an animal model. Urology. 2001;57:976–980.

[19] Gervais DA, McGovern FJ, Arellano RS, McDougal WS, Mueller PR. Renal cell carcinoma: clinical experience and technical success with radio-frequency ablation of 42 tumors. Radiology 2003;226:417-424.

[20] Goldberg SN, Solbiati L, Hahn PF, et al. Large-volume tissue ablation with radio frequency by using a clustered, internally cooled electrode technique: laboratory and clinical experience in liver metastases. Radiology 1998;209(2):371–379.

[21] Rehman J, Landman J, Lee D, Venkatesh R, Bostwick DG, Sundaram C, Clayman RV. Needle-based ablation of renal parenchyma using microwave, cryoablation, impedance- and temperature-based monopolar and bipolar radiofrequency, and liquid and gel chemoablation: laboratory studies and review of the literature. J Endourol. 2004 Feb;18(1):83-104.

[22] Farrell MA, Charboneau WJ, DiMarco DS, Chow GK, Zincke H, Callstrom MR, et al. Imaging-guided radiofrequency ablation of solid renal tumors. AJR Am J Roentgenol 2003;180:1509- 1513.

[23] Stern JM, Svatek R, Park S, Hermann M, Lotan Y, et al. Intermediate comparision of partial nephrectomy and radiofrequency ablation for clinical T1a renal tumors. BJUI. 2007; 100: 287-90.

[24] Stern Jm, Park S. Anderson K.Kidney tumor radiofrequency ablation: Experience in ASA I and ASA II patients. J Urol 2006.

[25] Goldberg SN, Hahn PF, Tanabe KK, Mueller PR, Schima W, Athanasoulis CA, et al. Percutaneous radiofrequency tissue ablation: does perfusion-mediated tissue cooling limit coagulation necrosis? J Vasc Interv Radiol 1998;9:101-111.

[26] Gervais DA, McGovern FJ, Arellano RS, McDougal WS, Mueller PR. Radiofrequency ablation of renal cell carcinoma: part 1, Indications, results, and role in patient management over a 6-year period and ablation of 100 tumors. AJR Am J Roentgenol. 2005 Jul;185(1):64-71.

[27] Zagoria RJ, Traver MA, Werle DM, Perini M, Hayasaka S, Clark PE. Oncologic efficacy of CT-guided percutaneous radiofrequency ablation of renal cell carcinomas. AJR Am J Roentgenol. 2007 Aug;189(2):429-36.

[28] Lucas SM, Stern JM, Adibi M, et al. Renal function outcomes in patients treated for renal masses smaller than 4 cm by ablative and extirpative techniques. J Urol 2008;179:75-80.

[29] Bensalah K, Zeltser I, Tuncel A, et al. Evaluation of costs and morbidity associated with laparoscopic radiofrequency ablation and laparoscopic partial nephrectomy for treat- ing small renal tumours. BJU Int 2007;101:467-71.

[30] Weight CJ, Kaouk JH, Hegarty NJ, et al. Correlation of radiographic imaging and histopathology following cryoablation and radio frequency ablation for renal tumors. J Urol 2008;179:1277-83.

[31] Breen DJ, Rutherford EE, Stedman B, et al. Management of renal tumors by image-guided radiofrequency ablation: experience in 105 tumors. Cardiovasc Intervent Radiol 2007;30:936-42.

[32] Traver MA, Werle DM, Clark PE, Zagoria PJ, Heilbrun ME, Hall MG. Oncological efficacy and factors influencing the success of computerized tomography (CT)-

guided percutaneous radiofrequency ablation (RFA) on renal neoplasm. J Urol 2006;175(Suppl):360.

[33] Matsumoto ED, Johnson DB, Ogan K, et al. Short-term efficacy of temperature-based radiofrequency ablation of small renal tumors. Urology 2005;65:877–81.

[34] Gallego Vilar D, José Povo Martin I, Miralles Aguado J, Garau Perelló C, Bosquet Sanz M, Gimeno Argente V, Cifrián M, García Vila J, Gallego Gómez J. Radiofrequency ablation as an alternative treatment for organ confined renal tumor.Actas Urol Esp. 2010 Nov;34(10):860-5.

[35] Bastide C, Garcia S, Anfossi E, et al. Histologic evaluation of radio- frequency ablation in renal cancer. Eur J Surg Oncol 2006;32:980–3. [58] Brausi M, Castagnetti G, Gavioli M, et al. Radiofrequency (rf) ablation of renal tumors does not produce complete tumor destruction: Results of a phase II study. Eur Urol 2004;3(Suppl):14–7).

[36] Klingler HC, Marberger M, Mauermann J, et al. 'Skipping' is still a problem with radiofrequency ablation of small renal tumors. BJU Int. 2007;99:998 -1001).

[37] Matin SF, Ahrar K, Cadeddu JA, et al. Residual and recur- rent disease following renal energy ablative therapy: a multi-institutional study. J Urol. 2006;176:1973-1977.

[38] Nguyen CT, Lane BR, Kaouk JH, Hegarty N, Gill IS, Novick AC, Campbell SC. Surgical salvage of renal cell carcinoma recurrence after thermal ablative therapy. J Urol. 2008 Jul;180(1):104-9; discussion 109.

[39] Janzen N, Zisman A, Pantuck AJ, Perry K, Schulam P, Belldegrun AS. Minimally invasive ablative approaches in the treatment of renal cell carcinoma. Curr Urol Rep 2002;3:13–20.

[40] Campbell SC, Novick AC, Herts B, et al. Prospective evalua- tion of fine needle aspiration of small, solid renal masses: accuracy and morbidity. Urology. 1997;50:25-29.

[41] Chawla SN, Crispen PL, Hanlon AL, Greenberg RE, Chen DY, Uzzo RG. The natural history of observed enhancing renal masses: meta-analysis and review of the world litera- ture. J Urol. 2006;175:425-431.

[42] Kunkle DA, Crispen PL, Chen DY, Greenberg RE, Uzzo RG. Enhancing renal masses with zero net growth during active surveillance. J Urol. 2007;177:849-854.

[43] Kunkle DA, Egleston BL, Uzzo RG. Excise, ablate or observe: the small renal mass dilemma—a meta-analysis and review. J Urol. 2008;179:1227-1233.

[44] Smaldone MC, Kutikov A, Egleston BL, Canter DJ, Viterbo R, Chen DY, Jewett MA, Greenberg RE, Uzzo RG. Small renal masses progressing to metastases under active surveillance: A systematic review and pooled analysis. Cancer. 2011 Jul 15. doi: 10.1002/cncr.26369.

[45] Gill IS, Remer EM, Hasan WA, et al. Renal cryoablation: outcome at 3 years. J Urol. 2005;173:1903-1907.

[46] Shingleton WB, Sewell PE Jr. Cryoablation of renal tumours in patients with solitary kidneys. BJU Int. 2003;92:237-239.

[47] Raman JD, Thomas J, Lucas SM, et al. Radiofrequency ablation for T1a tumors in a solitary kidney: promising in- termediate oncologic and renal function outcomes. Can J Urol. 2008;15:3980-3985.

[48] Jacobsohn KM, Ahrar K, Wood CG, Matin SF. Is radiofre- quency ablation safe for solitary kidneys? Urology. 2007; 69:819-823; discussion 823.

[49] Traver MA, Werle DM, Clark PE, Zagoria PJ, Heilbrun ME, Hall MG. Oncological efficacy and factors influencing the success of computerized tomography (CT)-guided percu- taneous radiofrequency ablation (RFA) on renal neo- plasm. J Urol 2006;175(Suppl):360.

[50] Weiser AZ, Raj G, O'Connel M, Robertson CN, Nelson RC, Polascik TJ. Complications after percutaneous radiofre- quency ablation of renal tumors. Urology 2005;66:1176–80.

[51] Clements T, Lin YK, Raman JD. Current status of ablative techniques for small renal masses Expert Rev Anticancer Ther. 2011 Jun;11(6):879-91.

[52] Hakimé A, Hines-Peralta A, Peddi H, et al. Combination of radiofrequency ablation with antiangiogenic therapy for tumor ablation efficacy: study in mice. Radiology 2007;244(2):464–470.

[53] Livraghi T, Goldberg SN, Lazzaroni S, et al. Hepatocellular carcinoma: radiofrequency ablation of medium and large lesions. Radiology 2000;214(3):761–768.

[54] Ahmed M, Liu Z, Humphries S, Goldberg SN. Computer modeling of the combined effects of perfusion, electrical conductivity, and thermal conductivity on tissue heating patterns in radiofrequency tumor ablation. Int J Hyperthermia 2008;24(7):577–588.

[55] Aubé C, Schmidt D, Brieger J, et al. Influence of NaCl concentrations on coagulation, temperature, and electrical conductivity using a perfusion radiofrequency ablation system: an ex vivo experimental study. Cardiovasc Intervent Radiol 2007;30(1):92–97.

[56] Rhim H, Dodd GD 3rd. Radiofrequency thermal ablation of liver tumors. J Clin Ultrasound 1999;27(5):221–229.

[57] Chen Q, Krol A, Wright A, Needham D, Dewhirst MW, Yuan F. Tumor microvascular permeability is a key determinant for antivascular effects of doxorubicin encapsulated in a temperature sensitive liposome. Int J Hyperthermia 2008; 24(6):475–482.

[58] Solazzo SA, Ahmed M, Schor-Bardach R, et al. Liposomal doxorubicin increases radiofrequency ablation-induced tumor destruction by increasing cellular oxidative and nitrative stress and accelerating apoptotic pathways. Radiology 2010;255(1):62–74.

[59] Bae Y, Buresh RA, Williamson TP, Chen TH, Furgeson DY. Intelligent biosynthetic nanobiomaterials for hyperthermic combination chemotherapy and thermal drug targeting of HSP90 inhibitor geldanamycin. J Control Release 2007;122(1):16–23.

[60] Algan O, Fosmire H, Hynynen K, et al . External beam radiotherapy and hyperthermia in the treatment of patients with locally advanced prostate carcinoma. Cancer 2000;89(2):399–403.

[61] Solazzo S, Mertyna P, Peddi H, Ahmed M, Horkan C, Goldberg SN . RF ablation with adjuvant therapy: comparison of external beam radiation and liposomal doxorubicin on ablation efficacy in an animal tumor model. Int J Hyperthermia 2008; 24(7):560–567.

[62] Horkan C, Dalal K, Coderre JA, et al. Reduced tumor growth with combined radiofrequency ablation and radiation therapy in a rat breast tumor model. Radiology 2005;235(1):81–8.

[63] Mayer R, Hamilton-Farrell MR, van der Kleij AJ, et al. Hyperbaric oxygen and radiotherapy. Strahlenther Onkol 2005;181(2):113–1.

7

Renal Tumors in Patients with von Hippel-Lindau Disease: "State of Art Review"

Mario Alvarez Maestro, Luis Martinez-Piñeiro and Emilio Rios Gonzalez
Hospital Universitario Infanta Sofia, Madrid
Spain

1. Introduction

The disease that has perpetuated the names of two prestigious European physicians, **Eugen von Hippel and Arvid Lindau**, is a familial syndrome characterised by the occurrence of highly vascular tumours in different organs[1]. Von Hippel-Lindau (VHL) disease is a rare, autosomal dominant genetic disease (Online Mendelian Inheritance in Man 193300) that is estimated to occur in 1/36,000 live births and with clinical manifestations usually becoming apparent between 18 and 30 years. VHL germline mutation predisposes patients to renal cysts and carcinoma, central nervous system and retina hemangioblastoma, pancreatic cysts and neuroendocrine tumors, pheochromocytoma, endolymphatic sac tumors and epididymal or adnexal cystadenoma[2]. Clinical diagnosis requires one major manifestation of von HippelLindau disease in patients with a familial history, and at least two major manifestations including one haemangioblastoma in isolated cases. Patients are at high risk for early multiple and recurrent clear cell Renal Cell Carcinoma (RCC) [3]. Total nephrectomy was systematically done in the past to prevent the risk of metastatic progression, which led to end stage renal disease requiring dialysis. Preserving normal renal parenchyma emerged as a major therapeutic goal in VHL cases. Since several groups reported that most RCC in VHL cases has low pathological grade, grows slowly and never becomes metastatic at less than 3 cm, in the early 1990s Nephron Sparing Surgery (NSS) was developed. The standard therapeutic procedure for RCC in VHL cases was to monitor small lesions by imaging and perform partial nephrectomy for any RCC that became 2.5 to 3 cm. During the last decade percutaneous ablative therapies, such as RFA and cryotherapy that were developed to treat localized RCC in select patients emerged as a novel nephron sparing therapy applicable to patients with VHL.

The worldwide von Hippel-Lindau Family Alliance greatly contributes to such dissemination by organising International Symposia once every 2 years which are an excellent opportunity for doctors, scientists, and affected individuals to meet and exchange information on fundamental and clinical **issues (http:// www.vhl.org)**[2].

2. Historical aspects

Although the contributions of von Hippel and Lindau were decisive, many others played an important part in the description of clinical manifestations, but not all can be cited (a complete history of von Hippel-Lindau disease is detailed in the articles from Melmon and

Rosen, Lamiell and colleagues, and Resche and colleagues)[4-6]. In 1872, Jackson first described a cerebellar haemangioblastoma, and retinal haemangioblastoma was described by Panas and Rémy in 1879[1].

The first recorded case of a probable patient with von Hippel-Lindau disease was a 35-year-old woman who died in 1864 with eye and brain tumours[7]. In 1895 von Hippel described the fundoscopic findings in the eye of a 23-year-old man, Otto Mayer, who had presented 2 years earlier with visual loss. Both the superior temporal artery and vein were dilated and supplied a prominent rounded mass located at the periphery of retina[8]. In 1904, von Hippel presented further details of the same patient, who had developed three similar lesions, as well as another similar case, of a 28-year-old man[9]. Von Hippel studied the histological characteristics of the right eye of Otto Mayer and concluded in 1911 that the retinal lesion was a congenital cystic capillary angiomatosis, which he named angiomatosis retinae[10]. However, it was Arvid Lindau who linked the retinal, cerebral, and visceral components of the disease into a single coherent entity in 1926. In his dissertation, he added 16 of his own patients to 24 previously reported patients with cystic cerebellar tumours[11]. He noted that cerebellar tumours were frequently associated with retinal lesions but also with renal cysts, hypernephroma (renal cell carcinoma), and pancreatic and epididymal cysts. The term von Hippel-Lindau disease was first used by Davison and colleagues[12] in 1936 and has been in common use since the 1970s. In 1964, Melmon and Rosen summarized these data and coined the term "von Hippel-Lindau disease"[4].

The most recent developments have followed the identification of the VHL gene, first located on 3p25–26 in 1988 by Seizinger and colleagues, and fully described in 1993 by Latif and coworkers[1, 3].

3. Genetic disorders and renal cell carcinoma

RCC represents 2-3% of all cancers, 7000 people are diagnosed with RCC each year in the UK, and 3600 annually succumb to the disease. It is estimated that 54,390 men and women in the United States will be diagnosed with kidney cancer, while 13,010 will die of their disease in next year. This number can also be expressed as 1 in 72 men and women will be diagnosed with cancer of the kidney during their lifetime and this incidence continues to rise[13].

There is an apparent increase in the incidence of RCC of 2.5% per year. This may in part be attributed to improved imaging techniques and an increased detection rate of incidental lesions.

Approximately 4% of RCCs are of hereditary origin and VHL is the commonest cause.

Furthermore, approximately 75% of RCCs are of clear cell histology (cRCC), and VHL is the hereditary cause of cRCC[14]. There are at least six other histological subtypes, each associated with a hereditary syndrome[15] (table 1). Hereditary cancer syndromes can be difficult to identify and early recognition is important, as it facilitates correct management of the patient, as well as screening of relatives. Principally, mutations can be "loss-of-function mutations" in tumor suppressor genes and "gain-of-function-mutations" in protooncogenes, which are then called oncogenes. Research regarding hereditary clear cell RCC has led to the identification of a relevant gene locus on the short arm of chromosome 3. This loss-off-function mutation led to the assumption of the existence of a tumor suppressor gene, and subsequently, further research led to the identification of the VHL gene.

Syndrome	Gene locations	Relative frequency	Histology	Other renal abnormalities	Systemic associations
VHL	3p26	28- 45%	Clear cell	Cysts	CNS haemangioblastoma Retinal angiomas Pancreatic cysts and neoplasm Phaeochromocytoma
Tuberous sclerosis	9q34, 16p13	1-2%	Clear cell	Cysts, papillary, oncocytoma	CNS tubers Cutaneous angiofibromas
Hereditary papillary RCC	7q34	19%	Papillary type 1	None	None known
Birt-Hogg- Dube	17p11	8-15%	Chromophobe	Clear cell, papillary, oncocytoma	Lung cysts Pneumothorax
Lynch type 2	2p16, 3p31	2-9%	Transitional cell carcinoma	None	Carcinoma of colon, ovary, endometrium, stomach
Medullary carcinoma of the kidney	11p	Unknown	Medullary carcinoma	None	Sickle cell trait
Hyperparathyroidism Jaw tumour	1q25	Unknown	Papillary	Cysts	Parathyroid tumours Fibro-osseous mandibular/ maxillary tumours
Familial papillary thyroid cancer	1q21	Unknown	Papillary	Oncocytoma	Papillary thyroid cancer Nodular thyroid disease

Table 1. The hereditary renal cancer syndromes

In the early 1980s, the search to identify a loss of heterozygosity in one of the alleles of a cancer gene was initiated, with the hope that loss of heterozygosity would indicate the presence of a cancer gene at that location. A tumor suppressor gene requires loss of function or inactivation of one or both of the genes, often by mutation of 1 allele combined with deletion, or loss, of the second allele, whereas, an oncogene is activated by 1 change in the gene. In the initial studies, loss of segments at chromosome 3 in tumor tissue suggested that a cancer gene for kidney cancer was present at this location[16]. Dr Knudson's "two hit" theory postulates that most tumor suppressor genes encode proteins responsible for the negative regulation of cellular growth. A mutation that causes a loss of the function in one these proteins will lead to tumorigenesis or uninhibited cell growth. As the gene of interest for clear cell kidney cancer was too large to localize with the technology that was available at the time, an approach focusing on a hereditary form of kidney cancer, von Hippel-

Lindau, was used as the model of investigation. The hope was that the gene involved in hereditary kidney cancer may involve the same gene as in the sporadic form of kidney cancer[17]. Lubensky and colleague performed a study that supported the two-hit theory of inheritance in VHL disease. The makeup of 26 renal cysts was studied with microdissection techniques. They found that each cyst was lined with a single layer of clear epithelial cells. Twenty-five of the 26 cysts had a mutation of the wild-type allele; in only one case was the usual heterozygosity of the disease maintained. This finding supports two-hit theory: once the heterozygosity for VHL is lost in a specific organ, in this case the kidney, the cyst can progress into a tumor[18].

4. Genetics in von Hippel-Lindau

Consistent loss of the short arm of chromosome 3 in VHL associated kidney tumors was identified[19]. Genetic linkage analysis was utilized to help identify the VHL gene, which was identified on the short arm of chromosome 3p[20]. The loss of the single normal allele of the VHL gene in the kidney cancer cell samples was critical and suggested that there was an inherited gene at this location, which was associated with the development of VHL-associated clear cell kidney cancer. Germline mutations on the VHL gene are identified in nearly 100% of VHL families[21]. The disease is caused by germline mutations in the VHL tumour-suppressor gene; the same gene is inactivated in most cases of sporadic renal-cell carcinoma and Central Nervous System (CNS) haemangioblastomas. The VHL gene seems to be pivotal in the processes of angiogenesis, an oxygensensing pathway involving the hypoxia-inducible factor (HIF), a heterodimeric transcription factor. The VHL gene product targets the subunit of HIF for polyubiquitylation and proteasomal degradation. This is the rationale for development of specific inhibitors of hypoxia-inducible factors and their downstream targets, which lead to potential new treatments. The development of a second mutation causing deletion of the normal VHL allele leads to tumor formation in affected individuals. More than 300 different types of mutations have been described that involve the three exons of the VHL gene.

The different clinical manifestations of VHL can be associated with the location and type of the VHL gene mutation[22, 23]. Penetrance of the traits is far from complete, and for some such as pheochromocytomas, they tend to be clustered in certain families but do not occur in others[24]. Maranchie et al.[25] identified a significantly higher incidence of renal cell carcinoma in patients with partial germline VHL mutations vs. those with complete VHL gene mutations. It is now known that with mutation analysis (e.g., insertion, deletion, missense, or nonsense) and the location (e.g., codon position) of the mutation, correlations can be made to the phenotype, i.e., the extent of involvement of the various organ systems affected by VHL.

Germline mutations in VHL have been identified in almost all patients with von Hippel-Lindau disease and correlations between the genotype and the phenotype are emerging, confirming clinical distinction based on the presence or absence of phaeochromocytoma. Such mutations have been identified in several patients without classic clinical criteria and a diagnosis of von Hippel-Lindau disease must now be considered in patients with an apparently sporadic tumour, especially in the case of phaeochromocytomas. Specific germline mutations in VHL have been associated with a rare recessive haematological condition (Chuvash polycythaemia) and might also be implicated in some sporadic apparently congenital polycythaemias[26].

The function of the VHL gene has been evaluated extensively. It is a small gene that encodes 854 nucleotides on 3 exons and is responsible for encoding the VHL protein[20]. The VHL protein forms a complex with proteins including elongin C, elongin B, and Cul-2[27-29] and targets the @ subunits of the hypoxia inducible factors, such as HIF-@ and HIF-2@, which are instrumental to ubiquitin mediated degradation[30]. There are multiple downstream genes, such as Glut 1 (glucose transport), vascular endothelial growth factor (VEGF, blood vessel growth), epidermal growth factor (EGF), transforming growth factor (TGF-@), for which HIF regulates. The expression of these genes increases in clear cell carcinoma when the VHL gene is inactivated (figure 1). Many of the receptors for HIF regulated genes are the targets for the new targeted therapeutic approaches for clear cell carcinoma[31]. Studies have shown that if the VHL complex is unable to bind to the HIF proteins, tumorigenesis results. Mutations in the oxygen-dependent domain or the VHL binding site of HIF-2-@, but not of HIF-1-@, result in tumorigenesis in xenograft models. Kondo and colleagues[33] showed that inhibition of only HIF-2-@ suppresses pVHL deficient tumor growth. This finding established that HIF-2-@ is a critical component to tumorigenesis in clear cell RCC. As previously discussed, HIF proteins are key regulators of oxygen homeostasis, and tight regulation of HIF allows cell survival and growth at the time of hypoxic stress. HIF acts via transcriptional regulation of VEGF, PDGF, EGFR, GLUT1, erythropoietin, and TGF-@. Loss of VHL is thought to result in a pseudohypoxic state, so that cellular response pathways mediated by HIF are activated despite normal oxygen conditions.

Understanding the VHL pathway and these pseudohypoxic pathways has provided the opportunity to develop therapies that target the downstream HIF pathway genes VEGF and PDGF with agents such as sunitinib that have a high affinity for the VEGF and PDGF receptors.

Other strategies, such as targeting HIF transcription and HIF stability, also are being evaluated in clinical trials.

5. Clinical diagnosis

VHL disease is among the group of disorders known as "phakomatoses" in which lesions arise from a single germ layer. The lesions of VHL disease are primarily mesodermal in origin. The clinical manifestations of VHL disease span a spectrum of phenotypic variability. It has virtually complete penetrance but variable expressivity. The syndrome is characterized by multiple tumor types, including kidney tumors, pheochromocytomas, epididymal cystadenomas, retinal angiomas, hemangiomas of the CNS, and pancreatic islet cell tumors.

Diagnosis of von Hippel-Lindau disease is often based on clinical criteria. Patients with a family history, and a CNS haemangioblastoma (including retinal haemangioblastomas), phaeochromocytoma, or clear cell renal carcinoma are diagnosed with the disease. Those with no relevant family history must have two or more CNS haemangioblastomas, or one CNS haemangioblastoma and a visceral tumour (with the exception of epididymal and renal cysts, which are frequent in the general population) to meet the diagnostic criteria[4, 34]. Specific correlations of genotype and phenotype have emerged in affected families. Several familial phenotypes of von Hippel-Lindau disease are now recognised, providing useful information to screen and counsel affected individuals. Type 1 families have a greatly reduced risk of phaeochromocytomas, but can develop all the other tumour types generally associated with the disease. Type 2 families have phaeochromocytomas, but have either a low-risk (type 2A) or high-risk (type 2B) for renal cell carcinomas. Type 2C families have phaeochromocytomas only, with no other neoplastic findings of VHL (table 2)[35].

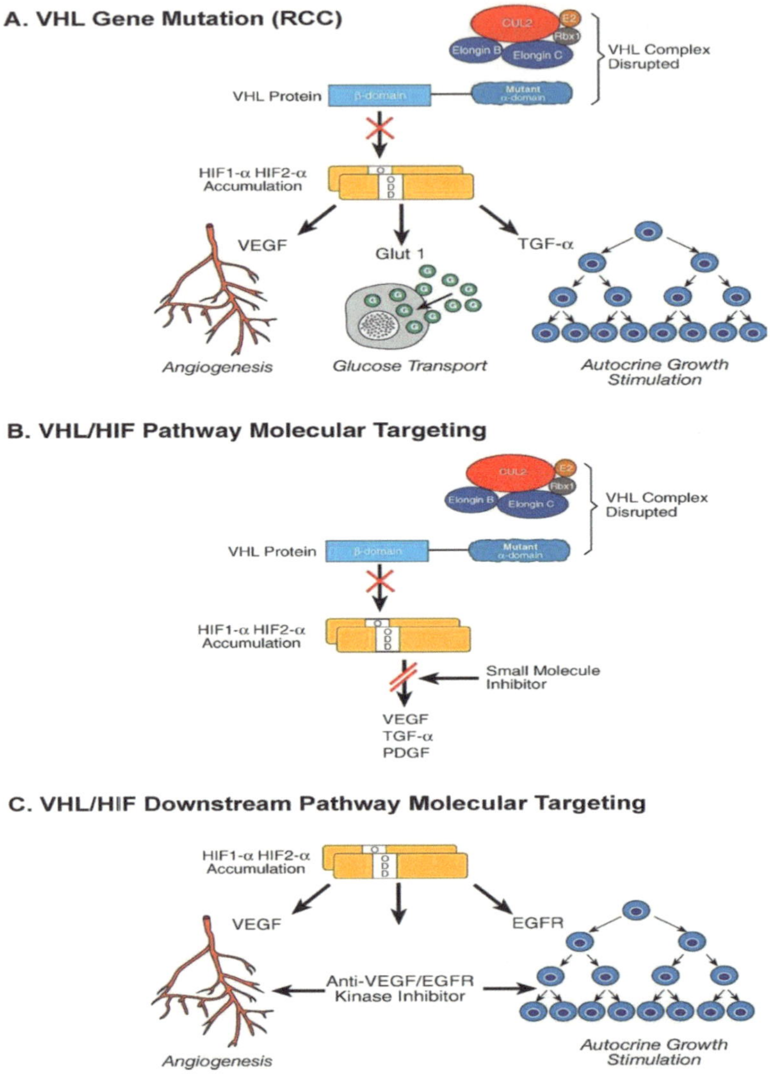

Fig. 1. [70] The *VHL* gene complex targets hypoxia-inducible factors (HIF) for ubiquitin-mediated degradation. When there is a mutation in the *VHL* gene in clear cell kidney cancer, in either the elongin binding or the HIF binding domain (A), HIF is not degraded and this protein over-accumulates. Increased HIF levels lead to increased transcription of a number of downstream pathway genes that are thought to be important in kidney cancer, such as vascular endothelial growth factor (VEGF), the glucose transporter, GLUT1, and transforming growth factor _ (TGF-@) (B). Targeted approaches to therapy currently include tyrosine kinase inhibitors that target the downstream gene receptors (C). Other approaches being developed to target the VHL-HIF pathway in clear cell kidney cancer include the development of small molecules or other agents which block HIF transcription. Reprinted from Linehan et al[32].

	Clinical characteristics
Type 1	Retinal haemangioblastomas CNS haemangioblastomas Renal cell carcinoma Pancreatic neoplasms and cysts
Type 2A	Phaeochromocytomas Retinal haemangioblastomas CNS haemangioblastomas
Type 2B	Phaeochromocytomas Retinal haemangioblastomas CNS haemangioblastomas Renal cell carcinomas Pancreatic neoplasms and cysts
Type 2C	Phaeochromocytoma only

*Endolymphatic sac tumours and cystadenomas of the epididymis and broad ligament have not been assigned to specific von Hippel-Lindau types.

Table 2. Genotype-phenotype classifications in families with von Hippel-Lindau disease*

The age of onset of VHL disease is variable and depends both on the expression of the disease within the individual and within the family and on the screening protocol used to detect asymptomatic lesions. More intensive screening regimens can increase greatly the number of affected individuals discovered in a family. Retinal lesions generally are the first lesions to be diagnosed.

Of the non-urologic stigmata, the most common in patients who survive to age 60 years are retinal angiomas, which affect 70% of patients, and CNS hemangiomas, which affect 84% of patients. The urologic manifestations include renal clear cell carcinoma (RCC), pheochromocytoma, and epididymal cystadenomas, which affect approximately 40%, 18%, and 10% of patients, respectively. Approximately a third of the patients who have VHL disease (13%-42%) die of metastatic disease.

The median age of death from VHL disease is 49 years, and the most common causes of death are neurologic complications of cerebellar haemangioblastoma and metastatic renal carcinoma. Approximately 53% of patients who have VHL disease die of complications of cerebellar hemangioblastoma, and 32% die of metastatic RCC[36].

6. Screening and surveillance for von Hippel-Lindau disease

Genetic testing for VHL is widely available and involves a simple blood test with an accuracy approaching 100% if the mutation is known[37]. However, the test is only available in select laboratories. Antenatal diagnosis is also feasible. In the past 15 years there have been major changes in the management of VHL. Better surveillance and genetic testing have improved detection rates of presymptomatic RCCs and these can now be treated with nephron-sparing procedures (NSS) before metastatic disease develops, preserving renal function as far as possible, but as yet there are no standardized screening protocols for VHL and guidelines vary between institutions.

The screening process for patients who have hereditary renal tumor syndromes developed at the Clinical Center of the National Institutes of Health (NIH) (table 3) includes karyotyping for the germline mutations of the VHL gene; abdominal CT with and without intravenous contrast material injection; renal ultrasound; ophthalmologic examination; brain, spinal, and internal auditory canal MRI; scrotal ultrasound for male patients; chest radiograph; and 24-hour urine and plasma catecholamines[38].

	PROTOCOL
Urinary catecholamines	From age 2 years: every 1-2 years
Opthalmoscopy	From infancy: yearly
Enhanced magnetic resonance imaging of brain and spine	From age 11: every 2 years From age 60: every 3-5 years
Abdominal computed tomography or ultrasound	From age 11: ultrasound yearly From age 20: computed tomography every 1-2 years

This is the protocol used at the National Institute of Health, USA.

Table 3. Screening of patients with Von Hippel- Lindau disease

The primary goals of preoperative evaluation for RCC are to define renal anatomy and to identify tumors in the brain, eye, pancreas, and adrenal glands that may present an intraoperative risk if undiagnosed. Such lesions include pheochromocytomas, which would require catecholamine blockade and probably resection at the time of renal surgery, and hemangioblastomas, which carry the risk of hemorrhage at the time of induction of anesthesia. Pancreatic neuroendocrine tumors also might be excised at a single surgical setting.

MRI can demonstrate CNS abnormalities most clearly while adequately imaging the abdominal viscera. CT, however, is the most accurate method of screening and follow-up for RCC. In addition to CT or MRI, an angiogram may be obtained preoperatively to define patient renal arterial anatomy before the first surgery. One study showed that angiogram identified only 16% of the multiple small renal tumors that were present [39], making it of limited utility beyond providing a vascular map for the first resection (but few hospitals perform this technique).

After surgical treatment for renal tumors, patients should be screened regularly to monitor for recurrence, metastasis, and loss of renal function. Periodic history and physical examination, routine laboratory screening tests, abdominal CT, renal ultrasound, chest CT or radiograph, and renal scans can be performed in addition to monitoring for new manifestations of VHL disease with periodic brain and spine MRIs, urinary catecholamines, and ophthalmologic evaluation[40].

Family members who carry a germline mutation but have not developed a tumour, and those with a mild phenotype can safely be imaged every 2-3 years. However, patients with mutations predisposing them to RCC should be assessed more frequently at 6-12 monthly intervals, depending on tumour growth rates[41]. Genetic testing can help predict the risk of developing RCC (as discussed above). Recent studies[42] have linked specific mutations to more aggressive forms of RCC and poorer survival rates. Such genetic stratification may allow more specific or patient focused surveillance in the future.

7. Renal cell carcinomas and renal cysts in von Hippel Lindau general features

Renal cell carcinomas are the major malignant neoplasm in von Hippel-Lindau disease and the primary cause of inherited renal cancer. These tumours are seen in 24–45% of patients, and adding renal cysts increases the finding of renal lesions to 60%. Renal disease is multicentric and bilateral in at least 75% of patients who have VHL disease. The mean age at presentation is 39 +/- 10 years, which is 10 to 20 years earlier than that reported for sporadic renal disease.

In addition to the young age of presentation, RCC associated with VHL disease also recurs frequently years. Although small renal tumours in this disease tend to be low grade and minimally invasive, their rate of growth varies widely[43]. Renal lesions are often multiple and bilateral. Walther and colleagues[44] estimated that 600 microscopic tumours and 1100 microscopic clear-cell-lined cysts might be present in the kidneys of some 37-year-old patients. Results of an investigation of 228 renal lesions in 28 patients, followed for at least 1 year, showed that transition from a cyst to a solid lesion was rare. Solid tumors in VHL disease have been observed to grow at rates of 0.2 to 2.2 cm/year (mean, 1.6 cm/year), which is somewhat faster than rates observed in sporadic RCC. The change that occurs in renal lesions over time in patients who have VHL disease is generally slow and constant, but it has been followed in only a small number of cases [45].

However, complex cystic and solid lesions can contain neoplastic tissue that frequently enlarges. Renal cell carcinomas often remain asymptomatic for long intervals. Thus, serial imaging of the kidneys is useful for early diagnosis. Occasionally, the more advanced cases with these neoplasms can present with haematuria, flank pain, or a flank mass. Renal cysts in von Hippel-Lindau disease are typically asymptomatic and seldom need treatment. Renal cysts are present in 59% to 63% of patients who have VHL disease, and some studies believe the number may be as high as 85% Cysts generally preceded the detection of solid tumors by about 3 to 7 years. Studies have shown that at least 21% of cystic renal lesions contain foci of RCC and RCC is reported to develop in 24% to 45% of patients who have VHL disease. Therefore, complex cysts need monitoring, as they often harbour solid components of renal cell carcinoma. Because of the frequent absence of early clinical symptoms and the importance of early detection, diagnosis during presymptomatic screening has the potential to enhance overall outcome.

Contrast-enhanced abdominal CT is the standard for detection of renal involvement in the disease. CT allows detection and quantification by size and number of renal cell carcinomas and cysts, allowing serial monitoring of individual lesions. Imaging is usually recommended in 3–5 mm sections, and before and after intravenous injection of contrast media. Precontrast and postcontrast MRI is an alternative method of detection for patients who have reduced renal function. These carcinomas are yellow or orange and are encapsulated. They can be solid or a mixture of solid and cystic in appearance. Histologically, they are always of the clear-cell subtype, and small carcinomas tend to be low grade. In addition, microscopic examination of small VHL renal lesions consistently demonstrated a pseudo-capsule surrounding these low-grade renal lesions. This pseudo-capsule has since proven to facilitate tumor resection by forming a natural tissue plane for dissection[46] . The recurrence rate of renal tumors is high in patients who have VHL disease. Examination of normal renal tissue of patients who have RCC and VHL disease has shown multiple microscopic renal tumors [43]. Treatment recommendations depend on tumour size.

8. Radiology of renal masses in VHL

RCC in VHL usually manifests as a complex cystic mass, which is also the most difficult type of renal lesion to accurately assess, especially when detected incidentally. The Bosniak classification was first described in 1986 and determines the management approach to the sporadic cystic renal mass[47]. The system was devised for CT but can also be applied to MRI. As some patients with VHL require long-term follow-up of renal manifestations with cross-sectional imaging, there are clear advantages of MRI, such as the absence of radiation. CNS manifestations are almost exclusively imaged with MRI in most institutions. MRI has also proved more accurate at assessing cystic pancreatic lesions and distinguishing phaeochromocytoma from adenoma on chemical shift imaging. It is also more sensitive than CT in detecting neuroendocrine tumours of the pancreas. For these reasons, several authors advocate annual surveillance of abdominal manifestations with MRI. These advantages must be weighed against potential risks of nephrogenic systemic fibrosis (NSF) with gadolinium compounds when used in renal impairment, as well as logistical factors, such as cost and limited access of MRI at some institutions. However, patients undergoing a lifetime of screening may accumulate relatively large doses of radiation to the kidneys as a consequence of annual screening with CT. Thus, there is no clear-cut answer which is the best imaging modality[48].

Before CT was widely available 13-42% of patients with VHL died of metastatic RCC[43]. The discovery of the VHL gene in 1993 unlocked a better understanding of the pathways involved in tumourigenesis. Surgery is still the only curative treatment of RCC. Bilateral nephrectomy with renal-replacement therapy would eradicate all tissue at risk for developing RCC and is a theoretical, but radical, option in a patient with VHL. However, patients with VHL do worse on renal-replacement therapy. A large study[49] showed a 5-year survival rate of 65% in VHL patients on dialysis compared with 71-86% for the non-VHL group. But renal impairment in the absence of renal surgery is rare among VHL patients. As patients with VHL do worse with renal- replacement therapy, the aim of successful management is to preserve renal function balanced against the risk of developing renal metastatic disease. The secondary aim is to minimize the number of procedures performed to accomplish this. To accomplish these aims accurate imaging-guided diagnosis and nephron-sparing procedures are important.

9. Nephron-sparing surgery and other treatments in von Hippel-Lindau disease

RCC in von Hippel-Lindau disease differs from its sporadic counterpart in that the diagnosis is made at a young age, and there are usually multiple bilateral renal tumors. Although these are generally low-stage tumors, they are capable of progression with metastasis and represent a frequent cause of death in patients with von Hippel-Lindau disease. RCC in these patients is characterized histopathologically by both solid tumors and renal cysts that contain either frank carcinoma or a lining of hyperplastic clear cells representing incipient carcinoma.

Therefore, adequate surgical treatment of localized RCC in vonHippel-Lindau disease requires excision of all solid and cystic renal lesions. Choyke et al.[50] have shown that intraoperative ultrasonography may be a valuable adjunct for this population of patients. In their series, this study identified additional tumors in 25% of patients with hereditary renal cancer undergoing renal exploration.

The surgical options in patients with bilateral RCC and von Hippel-Lindau disease are bilateral nephrectomy and renal replacement therapy or partial nephrectomy to avoid end-stage renal failure. The general philosophy has been to pursue nephron-sparing surgery if possible, given the multifocal nature of the disease, even for centrally located tumors. The treatment options for patients who have renal involvement in VHL disease have evolved during the last 3 decades. Staged bilateral nephrectomy and hemodialysis have progressed to partial nephrectomy and NSS. The best management approach for VHL disease balances the goals of minimizing the risk of RCC metastasis and preserving renal function and attempts to minimize the total number of surgeries a patient will require over a lifetime[51] . There are no specific guidelines regarding the type or timing of surgery in patients who have VHL disease.

The treatment strategy of total nephrectomy and Renal Replacement Theraphy (RRT) removes all the tissue at risk for RCC and, with it, the risk of metastases. Goldfarb and colleagues[52] noted a 5-year survival rate of 65% in patients who had VHL disease and who were treated with bilateral nephrectomy and RRT. Some transplant centers consider the presence or potential for VHL-related tumors, including renal and extrarenal tumors, a contraindication for renal transplantation.

The indications for NSS are localized malignancy in a solitary kidney, bilateral synchronous renal lesions, and renal tumors in patients whose contralateral kidney is threatened by local, systemic, or genetic risk factors[53].

Although early results of partial nephrectomy were promising, subsequent studies suggested a high incidence of postoperative tumour recurrence in the remaining portion of the kidney. It is likely that most of these local recurrences were a manifestation of residual microscopic RCC that was not removed at the time of the original partial nephrectomy. Walther and colleagues[54] have reported extensively on their approach of enucleation of small renal tumors associated with VHL disease (figure 2). Preservation of the perirenal fat and fascia are believed to be important in improving the patient's ability to undergo subsequent renal surgeries. The renal capsule is incised, circumscribing the lesions to be resected. All cystic lesions are excised, if possible, because of the potential for development of RCC[46]. Smaller cystic lesions are unroofed, and the base is fulgurated (however it has not been shown that this is completely safe).

A study from the NIH[55] showed that renal tumors less than 3 cm in size are not considered an indication for radical surgery. Patients who have VHL disease generally are followed expectantly until solid renal lesions are larger than 3 cm in diameter. In the previously mentioned NIH study, the 3-cm threshold for surgery was evaluated in 52 patients who had VHL disease. None of these patients had metastatic disease, and none required RRT. Forty-six of these patients underwent NSS rather than radical nephrectomy. Forty-four patients who had VHL disease developed renal tumors larger than 3 cm. From this study, the authors concluded that using a 3-cm tumor diameter as a threshold for NSS may help prevent metastatic disease. These authors also noted the importance of intraoperative Doppler ultrasound for locating tumors and verifying that all tumors have been removed[56]. A follow-up of this study[38] revealed that metastasis did not develop in any patient who had a solid renal tumor smaller than 3 cm. Of 50 patients who had RCC, metastasis developed in 1 patient who had a primary renal tumor that was 4.5 cm in greatest diameter.

One multicenter study[57] delineated the long-term outcomes after surgical treatment of localized RCC in 65 patients with von Hippel-Lindau disease managed at eight medical centers in the United States. RCC was present bilaterally and unilaterally in 54 and 11 patients, respectively. Radical nephrectomy and partial nephrectomy were performed in 16 and 49 patients, respectively. The mean postoperative follow-up interval was 68 months. The 5-year and 10-year cancer-specific survival rates for all patients were 95% and 77%, respectively. The corresponding rates for patients treated with partial nephrectomy were 100% and 81%, respectively. In the latter group, 25 patients (51%) developed postoperative local recurrence; however, only two of these patients had concomitant metastatic disease. Survival free of local recurrence was 71% at 5 years but only 15% at 10 years. Only 2 of 25 patients who had local recurrence after NSS had metastatic disease at the time recurrence was detected.

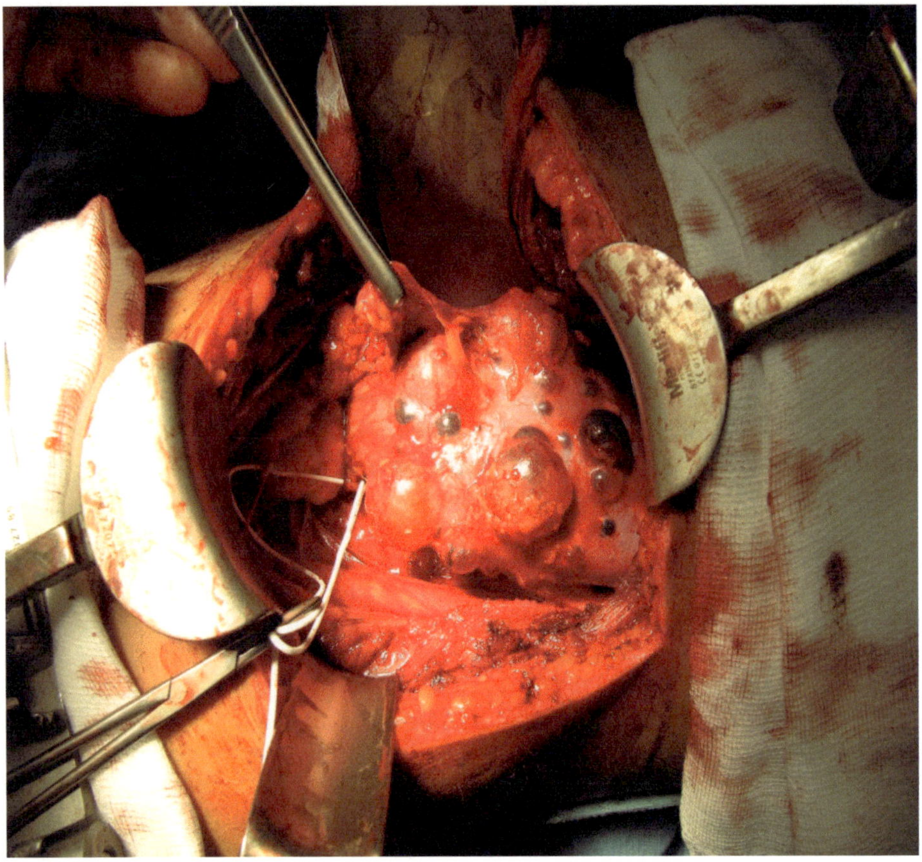

Fig. 2. Intraoperative photograph of multiple tumors and cysts in the kidney in a patient who has VHL disease.

Similarly, Roupret et al.[58] reported a 27.4% incidence of local recurrence at mean follow-up of 55.9 months after partial nephrectomy for patients with von Hippel-Lindau disease, confirming that these patients are at much higher risk for local recurrence than are patients with sporadic RCC. Ploussard and colleagues[59] published a series to evaluate the risks of local recurrence after NSS in patients who have VHL disease. Seventeen of 21 patients underwent surgery for RCC when tumors reached 3 cm. Eight patients developed a recurrence, and the mean time to local recurrence was 53+/- 38.8 months (range, 10–115 months). The disease-specific survival rate was 93.8% at 10 years. No metastasis or chronic renal insufficiency was observed in patients undergoing NSS only.

Taken together, these studies suggest that partial nephrectomy can provide effective initial treatment of patients with RCC and von Hippel-Lindau disease but should be withheld until tumor size reaches or eclipses 3.0 cm. Studies show that up to 85% of patients who have VHL disease experience de novo renal tumor recurrence at 10 years[57].

After nephron-sparing surgery, patients with von Hippel-Lindau disease must be observed closely because most will eventually develop locally recurrent RCC with the concomitant need for repeated renal surgery. In this setting, repeated partial nephrectomy can be challenging because of postoperative fibrosis, and some centers are moving toward thermal ablative modalities to reclaim local control and many surgeons are reluctant to perform additional NSS because of complications related to postoperative fibrosis[60]. These salvage surgeries were greatly complicated by severe fibrosis, scarring, and the obliteration of normal anatomic planes. The authors concluded that aggressive surgical intervention in these patients is indicated, because none of the patients developed metastatic disease as long as 7 years after surgery, and there was 100% survival in this cohort[61]. NSS has been performed using the laparoscopic approach in select centers, but the inability to achieve reliable hypothermia along with prolonged ischemia times and increased complication rates have limited in its widespread application. **At present, open NSS should be considered the standard of care for treating RCC in the setting of VHL disease**.

When removal of all renal tissue is necessary to achieve control of malignant disease, renal transplantation can provide satisfactory replacement therapy for end-stage renal disease and appears to be safe despite the tumor diathesis.

Newer, minimally invasive techniques[62], such as radiofrequency ablation and cryoablation, have been applied recently as an alternative to excisional NSS in patients who have RCC. Ablative techniques may[63, 65] be performed by laparoscopic and percutaneous image-guided techniques. Jolly et al.[64] concluded in a recent published article that renal survival in patients with VHL who are treated for RCC has improved with time. Their renal survival curves actually reflect the decreasing need to remove all renal tissue to achieve local control of malignancy, in parallel with improved NSS and the emergence of renal salvage techniques such as Radio Frecuency Ablation (RFA) (figure 3a and 3b). As well as surgery, nephron sparing procedures now include RFA and cryoablation. In their experience since 2004 RFA has become the exclusive salvage technique. Overall a third of RFA sessions were performed in single functioning kidneys, including 8 in a total of 8 patients who had already been operated on twice and were not candidates for additional NSS.

These all have a role in the surgical management of VHL-associated RCC and experience of these newer modalities in VHL is increasing, and good preliminary success rates are being published. A small study by Shingleton and Sewell[66] reported the successful treatment of five small RCCs in four patients with VHL using MRI-guided cryoablation, but greater evidence is available for imaging- guided RFA treatment of RCCs in the context of VHL, demonstrating good success rates for exophytic tumours of up to 5 cm in size[67, 68].

In conclusion[69], as patients with VHL with RCC are increasingly treated with nephron sparing techniques, especially RFA, it must be remembered that only long-term follow-up can hopefully confirm that no unexpected metastasis develops beyond increased renal survival. In patients who have a single kidney or multiple bilateral lesions, collateral damage to normal renal parenchyma must be considered. For patients who have VHL disease, and all patients who have hereditary cancer syndromes, the goal of treatment is cancer control, not cancer cure, and preservation of functional parenchyma to avoid the morbidity associated with renal or adrenal loss.

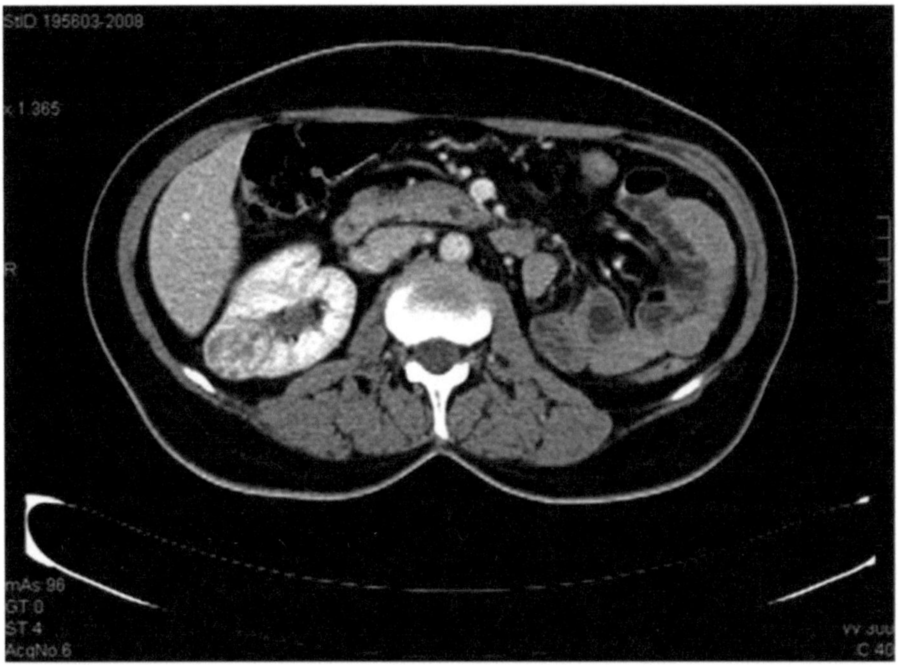

Fig. 3a. Renal tumor in a patient with solitary right kidney and VHL disease

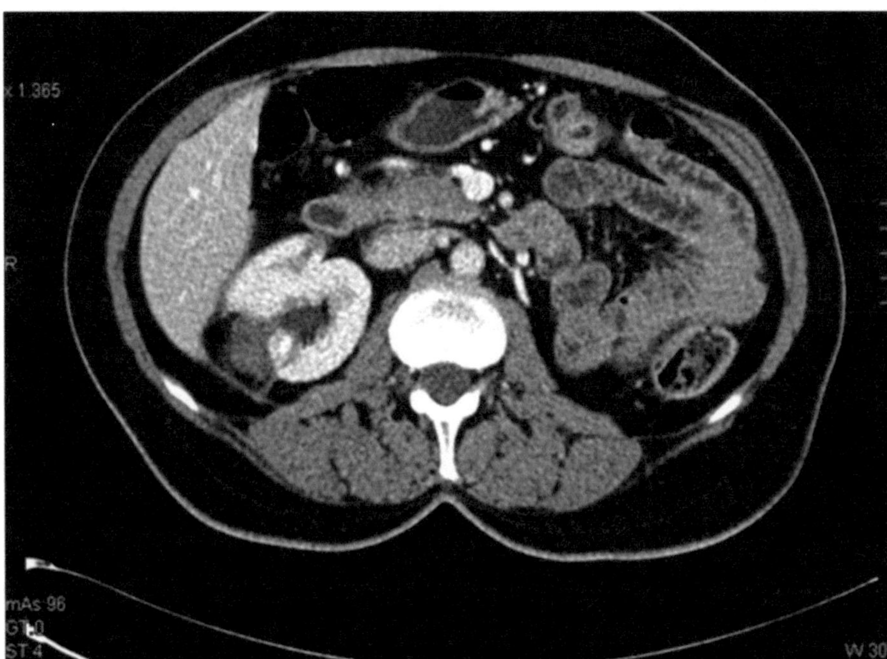

Fig. 3b. Contrast enhanced CT scan after radiofrequency ablation show the absence of contrast enhancement in the ablated area.

10. References

[1] Lonser RR, Glenn G, Walther McC, et al. Von-Hippel-Lindau disease. Lancet 2003, 361: 2059-67.

[2] Richard S, Graff J, Lindau J, Resche F. Von Hippel-Lindau disease. The Lancet, Volume 363, Issue 9416, 10 April 2004, Pages 1231-1234.

[3] Kaelin WG Jr. Molecular basis of the VHL hereditary cancer syndrome. Nat Rev Cancer 2003; 2: 673–82.

[4] Melmon KL, Rosen SW. Lindau's disease. Review of the literature and study of large kindred. Am J Med 1964, 36: 595–617.

[5] Lamiell JM, Salazar FG, Hsia YE. Von Hippel-Lindau disease affecting 43 members of single kindred. Medicine 1989; 68: 1–29.

[6] Resche F, Moisan JP, Mantoura J, et al. Hemangioblastomas, hemangioblastomatosis and von Hippel-Lindau disease. Adv Techn Stand Neurosurg 1993; 20: 197–303.

[7] Galezowski X, Traité iconographique d'opthalmoscopie. In: Baillière, ed. Diagnostic et traitement desaffections occulaires par les docteurs. Paris, Baillières, 1986.

[8] von Hippel E. Vorstellung eines Patienten mit einer sehr ungewöhnlichen Netzhaut. XXIV Verstellung der ophthalmologischen Gesellschaft (Heidelberg, 1895), JF Bergmann Verlag, Wiesbaden, 1896: 269.

[9] von Hippel E. Ueber eine sehr seltene Erkrankung der Netzhaut. Klinische Beobachtungen. A von Graefe's Arch Ophthalmol 1904; 59: 83–106.

[10] von Hippel E. Die anatomische Grundlage der von mir beschriebenen "sehr seltene Erkrankung der Netzhaut". *A von Graefe's Arch Ophthalmol* 1911; 79: 350–77.

[11] Lindau A. Studien über Kleinhirnzysten. Bau, Pathogenese und Beziehungen zur Angiomatosis retinae. Acta Pathol Microbiol Scand 1926; S1: 1–128.

[12] Davison C, Brock S, Dyke CG. Retinal and central nervous hemangioblastomatosis with visceral changes (von Hippel-Lindau's disease). Bull Neurol Instit NY 1936; 5: 72–93.

[13] SEER Cancer Statistics Review, 1975–2005. NCI 2007; (November 2007 SEER data submission. Available from URL:

[14] http://seer. cancer.gov/csr/1975_2005/results_merged/sect_01_overview.pdf and http://seer.cancer.gov/csr/1975_2005/results_merged/sect_11_ kidney_pelvis.pdf).

[15] Pavlovich CP, Schmidt LS. Searching for the hereditary causes of renal-cell carcinoma. Nat Rev Cancer 2004; 4: 381- 93.

[16] Choyke PL, Glenn GM, Walther MM, et al. Hereditary renal cancers. Radiology 2003; 226:33-46.

[17] Zbar B, Brauch H, Talmadge C, et al. Loss of alleles of loci on the short arm of chromosome 3 in renal cell carcinoma. Nature 1987; 327: 721- 4.

[18] Knudson AG. Genetics of human cancer. Annu Rev Genet 1986; 20: 231–51.

[19] Lubensky IA, Gnarra JR, Bertheau P, et al. Allelic deletions of the VHL gene detected in multiple microscopic clear cell renal lesions in von Hippel-Lindau disease patients. Am J Pathol 1996; 149(6):2089–94.

[20] Tory K, Brauch H, Linehan WM, et al. Specific genetic change in tumors associated with von Hippel-Lindau disease. J Natl Cancer Inst 1989; 81:1097–10.

[21] Latif F, Tory K, Gnarra JR, et al. Identification of the von Hippel-Lindau disease tumor suppressor gene. Science 1993; 260:1317–20.

[22] Stolle C, Glenn GM, Zbar B, et al. Improved detection of germline mutations in the von Hippel-Lindau disease tumor suppressor gene. Hum Mutat 1998; 12:417–23.

[23] Chen F, Kishida T, Yao M, et al. Germline mutations in the von Hippel-Lindau disease tumor suppressor gene: correlations with phenotype. Hum Mutat 1995; 5:66 –75

[24] Ong KR, Woodward ER, Killick P, et al. Genotype-phenotype correlations in von Hippel-Lindau disease. Hum Mutat 2007; 28:143–9.

[25] Neumann HPH, Zbar B. Renal cysts, renal cancer, and von Hippel-Lindau disease. Kidney Int 1997; 51:16 -26.

[26] Maranchie JK, Afonso A, Albert PS, et al. Solid renal tumor severity in von Hippel Lindau disease is related to germline deletion length and location. Hum Mutat 2004; 23:40–6.

[27] Ang SO, Chen H, Hirota K, et al. Disruption of oxygen homeostasis underlies congenital Chuvash polycythemia. *Nat Genet* 2002; 32: 614–21.

[28] Duan DR, Pause A, Burgess WH, et al. Inhibition of transcription elongation by the VHL tumor suppressor protein. Science 1995; 269: 1402–6.

[29] Kibel A, Iliopoulos O, DeCaprio JA, et al. Binding of the von Hippel-Lindau tumor suppressor protein to Elongin B and C. Science 1995;269:1444–6.

[30] Pause A, Lee S, Worrell RA, et al. The von Hippel-Lindau tumor suppressor gene product forms a stable complex with human CUL-2, a member of the Cdc53 family of proteins. Proc Natl Acad Sci USA 91997; 4:2156–61.

[31] Iliopoulos O, Jiang C, Levy AP, et al. Negative regulation of hypoxiainducible genes by the von Hippel-Lindau protein. Proc Natl Acad Sci USA 1996; 93:10595–9.

[32] Linehan WM. Editorial: Kidney Cancer, a Unique Opportunity for the Development of Disease Specific Therapy. J Urol 2002; 168: 2411–2.

[33] Linehan WM, Zbar B. Focus on kidney cancer. Cancer Cell 2004; 6: 223–8.

[34] Kondo K, Klco J, Nakamura E, Lechpammer M, Kaelin WG Jr. Inhibition of HIF is necessary for tumour suppression by the von Hippel-Lindau protein. Cancer Cell 2002; 1: 237–46.

[35] Escourolle R, Poirer J. Manual of Neuropathology. 2nd edn. Philadelphia: WB Saunders, 1978: 49–51.

[36] Hes F, Zewald R, Peeters T, et al. Genotype-phenotype correlations in families with deletions in the von Hippel-Lindau (VHL) gene. *Hum Genet* 2000; 106: 425–31.

[37] Martz CH. Von Hippel-Lindau disease: a genetic condition predisposing tumor formation. Oncol Nurs Forum 1991; 18(3):545–51.

[38] Linehan WM, Walther MM, Zbar B. The genetic basis of cancer of the kidney. J Urol 2003; 170:2163- 72.

[39] Herring JC, Enquist EG, Chernoff A, et al. Parenchymal sparing surgery in patients with hereditary renal cell carcinoma: 10-year experience. J Urol 2001; 165(3):777–81.

[40] Miller DL, Choyke PL, Walther MM, et al. von Hippel-Lindau disease: inadequacy of angiography for identification of renal cancers. Radiology 1991; 179(3):833–6.

[41] Maher ER, Yates JR, Harries R, et al. Clinical features and natural history of von Hippel-Lindau disease. Q J Med 1990; 77(283):1151–63.

[42] Choyke PL, Glenn GM, Walther MM, et al. von Hippel- Lindau disease: genetic, clinical, and imaging features. Radiology 1995; 194: 629- 42.

[43] Israel GM, Hindman N, Bosniak MA. Evaluation of cystic renal masses: comparison of CT and MR imaging by using the Bosniak classification system. Radiology 2004; 231:365- 71.

[44] Walther MM, Choyke PL, Glenn G, et al. Renal cancer in families with hereditary renal cancer: prospective analysis of a tumor size threshold for renal parenchymal sparing surgery. J Urol 1999; 161(5):1475–9.

[45] Walther MM, Lubensky IA, Venzon D, Zbar B, Linehan WM. Prevalence of microscopic lesions in grossly normal renal parenchyma from patients with von Hippel-Lindau disease, sporadic renal cell carcinoma and no renal disease: clinical implications. *J Urol* 1995; 154: 2010–14.

[46] Choyke PL, Glenn GM, Walther MM, et al. The natural history of renal lesions in von Hippel-Lindau disease: a serial CT study in 28 patients. AJR Am J Roentgenol 1992; 159(6):1229–34.

[47] Poston CD, Jaffe GS, Lubensky IA, et al. Characterization of the renal pathology of a familial form of renal cell carcinoma associated with von Hippel-Lindau disease: clinical and molecular genetic implications. J Urol 1995; 153(1):22–6.

[48] Bosniak MA. The current radiological approach to renal cysts. Radiology 1986; 158:1-10.

[49] Meister M., Choyke P., Anderson C., Patel U. Radiological evaluation, management, and surveillance of renal masses in Von Hippel–Lindau disease. Clinical Radiology, Volume 64, Issue 6, June 2009, Pages 589-600.

[50] Grubb 3rd RL, Choyke PL, Pinto PA, et al. Management of von Hippel- Lindau associated kidney cancer. Nat Clin Pract Urol 2005; 2: 248- 55.

[51] Choyke PL, Pavlovich CP, Daryanani KD, et al: Intraoperative ultrasound during renal parenchymal sparing surgery for hereditary renal cancers: A 10 year experience. J Urol 2001; 165:397-400.

[52] Fetner CD, Barilla DE, Scott T, et al. Bilateral renal cell carcinoma in von Hippel- Lindau syndrome: treatment with staged bilateral nephrectomy and hemodialysis. J Urol 1977; 117(4): 534–6.

[53] Goldfarb DA, Neumann HP, Penn I, et al. Results of renal transplantation in patients with renal cell carcinoma and von Hippel-Lindau disease. Transplantation 1997; 64(12):1726–9.

[54] Duffey BG, Choyke PL, Glenn G, et al. The relationship between renal tumor size and metastases in patients with von Hippel-Lindau disease. J Urol 2004; 172(1): 63–5.

[55] Walther MM, Thompson N, Linehan W. Enucleation procedures in patients with multiple hereditary renal tumors. World J Urol 1995; 13(4):248–50.

[56] Walther MM, Choyke PL, Glenn G, et al. Renal cancer in families with hereditary renal cancer: prospective analysis of a tumor size threshold for renal parenchymal sparing surgery. J Urol 1999; 161(5):1475–9.

[57] Walther MM, Choyke PL, Hayes W, et al. Evaluation of color Doppler intraoperative ultrasound in parenchymal sparing renal surgery. J Urol 1994; 152(6 Pt 1): 1984–7.

[58] Steinbach F, Novick AC, Zincke H, et al. Treatment of renal cell carcinoma in von Hippel- Lindau disease: a multicenter study. J Urol 1995; 153(6):1812–6.
[59] Roupret M, Hopirtean V, Mejean A, et al. Nephron sparing surgery for renal cell carcinoma and von Hippel-Lindau's disease: a single center experience. J Urol 2003; 170(5):1752–5.
[60] Ploussard G, Droupy S, Ferlicot S, et al. Local recurrence after nephron-sparing surgery in von-Hippel-Lindau disease. Urology 2007; 70(3):435–9.
[61] Bratslavsky G, Liu JJ, Ferlicot S, et al. Salvage partial nephrectomy for hereditary renal cancer: feasibility and outcomes. J Urol 2008; 179(1):67–70.
[62] Thompson RH, Leibovich BC, Lohse CM, et al. Complications of contemporary open nephron sparing surgery: a single institution experience. J Urol 2005; 174(3):855–8.
[63] Kunkle DA, Egleston BL, Uzzo RG. Excise, ablate or observe: the small renal mass dilemma-a meta-analysis and review. J Urol 2008; 179(4):1227–33.
[64] Aron M, Gill IS. Minimally invasive nephron-sparing surgery (MINSS) for renal tumours. Part II: probe ablative therapy. Eur Urol 2007; 51(2):348–57.
[65] Joly D., Méjean A. , Corréas J-M et al. Progress in Nephron Sparing Therapy for Renal Cell Carcinoma and von Hippel-Lindau Disease. The Journal of Urology, Volume 185, Issue 6, June 2011, Pages 2056-2060.
[66] Hwang JJ, Walther MM, Pautler SE et al: Radio frequency ablation of small renal tumors: intermediate results. J Urol 2004; 171: 1814.
[67] Shingleton WB, Sewell Jr PE. Percutaneous renal cryoablation of renal tumors in patients with von Hippel-Lindau disease. J Urol 2002; 167:1268-70.
[68] Gervais DA, McGovern FJ, Arellano RS, et al. Renal cell carcinoma: clinical experience and technical success with radio- frequency ablation of 42 tumors. Radiology 2003; 226: 417-24.
[69] Su LM, Jarrett TW, Chan DY, et al. Percutaneous computed tomography-guided radiofrequency ablation of renal masses in high surgical risk patients: preliminary results. Urology 2003; 61(Suppl. 1):26-33.
[70] Beth Reed A., Parekh D. Surgical Management of von Hippel-Lindau Disease: Urologic Considerations. Surgical Oncology Clinics of North America - Volume 18, Issue 1 (January 2009) (157-174).
[71] Rosner I, Bratslavsky G., Pinto P., Linehan W. The clinical implications of the genetics of renal cell carcinoma. Urologic Oncology: Seminars and Original Investigations, Volume 27, Issue 2, March-April 2009, Pages 131-136.

8

Exploitation of Aberrant Signalling Pathways as Useful Targets for Renal Clear Cell Carcinoma Therapy

Carol O'Callaghan and Orla Patricia Barry
University College Cork
Ireland

1. Introduction

Renal cell carcinoma (RCC) is the third leading cause of death among urological tumours, annually afflicts about 150, 000 people globally and causes nearly 78, 000 deaths (Jemal et al., 2008; Zbar et al., 2003). RCC is an epithelial tumour consisting of several different histological subtypes of which clear cell RCC is the prototypical. Traditionally treatment has been via surgery and immunotherapy. Surgical resection is appropriate for some patient cohorts including those with isolated metastases. However, recurrence is common even when the primary and metastatic sites have been aggressively resected (Couillard & deVere White, 1993). RCC is highly unresponsive to standard chemotherapy and the use of cytokine therapy with interleukin (IL)-2 or interferon (IFN)-α is associated with low rates of response and high rates of toxicity (Oudard et al., 2007). Thus, development of new therapies continues to be crucial to improve outcomes in patients with RCC.

The increased understanding of the molecular structure and aberrant activity of signalling pathways in RCC has lead to a flurry of research activity in the arena of targeted therapies namely anti-angiogenic vascular endothelial growth factor (VEGF) and the mammalian target of rapamycin (mTOR), both of which are involved in the pathogenesis of RCC (Mulders, 2009). These advancements in an obvious therapeutic gap have significantly improved the progression free survival (PFS) of patients with RCC. Despite the explosion in drug development during the past five years, however, PFS for patients with metastatic RCC (mRCC) still remains poor as none of the current targeted therapies possess the capacity to induce remission. In addition these drugs provide dose-limiting toxic side effects and so we are still faced with a considerable task in developing newer safer therapeutics for use as either first line agents or in combination with existing ones.

2. Targeted therapy for RCC

As the understanding of the molecular biology underlying RCC has increased, various components of growth and angiogenic signal transduction pathways have been identified as rational targets for therapeutic intervention in the treatment of patients with RCC and mRCC. The VEGF/VEGF receptor (VEGFR) pathway is one such target. VEGF expression is induced under hypoxic conditions triggering several mechanisms that promote angiogenesis (Ellis & Hicklin, 2008). Members of the VEGF family namely VEGF-A, -B, -C and -D regulate angiogenesis through binding to the related family of receptor tyrosine kinases (RTKs): VEGF receptors (VEGFR)-1, -2 and -3. The VEGFR consists of an extracellular ligand binding site, a transmembrane α-helical domain and an intracellular protein-tyrosine kinase region. Once activated, phosphorylated tyrosine residues on these receptor kinases provide high-affinity binding sites for components of the Raf/MEK/ERK (MAP Kinase) and PI3K/AKT signalling pathways which mediate cell growth and angiogenesis. Inhibition of the pathway involving VEGF-A activation of VEGFR-2 has undergone the most extensive investigation in recent years. This pathway mediates the formation and preservation of the blood vessel network which is vital for tumour cell survival and proliferation (Casanovas et al., 2005). In RCC, VEGF is also a powerful tumour growth factor. RCCs over-express the different VEGFRs and also produce as paracrine and autocrine growth factors, large amounts of VEGF (Qian et al., 2009). In tumours the VEGF isoforms -C and -D have been shown to activate the VEGFR3 receptor and to initiate the development and maintenance of a lymphatic system (He et al., 2005). Targeting this process in cancer treatment is now in the early stages of development. Presently, different therapeutic avenues exist for inhibiting the activation of receptor tyrosine kinases (RTKs). Monoclonal antibodies (mAbs) against growth factor ligands, or antibody fragments against RTK ligand-binding domain, can prevent binding of growth factors, thus attenuating RTK activity. Alternatively, the protein kinase can be targeted. Drugs that bind reversibly to the ATP-binding site within the kinase domain or to a small pocket that is immediately adjacent to the ATP-binding site are used to block the enzymatic activity of the kinase. Due to similarities within the amino acid structure of the kinase domain, ATP-competitive inhibitors can have cross reactivity with other structurally related kinases.

2.1 VEGF- antibody therapy/ligand competitors

2.1.1 Bevacizumab

Bevacizumab is an i.v. administered humanized monoclonal IgG1 antibody that targets and neutralises all major isoforms of circulating VEGF (Presta et al., 1997). By binding with high affinity to VEGF, bevacizumab inhibits its interaction with tyrosine kinase receptors thereby preventing the initiation of an angiogenic signal (Figure 1). This weakens existing microvasculature and production of new vasculature is inhibited. The loss of vascularisation eventually leads to tumour cell death (Jain, 2005).

Bevacizumab is used in the treatment of a wide range of cancer types including RCC, colon, brain and lung cancers. It was approved in 2009 for the first-line treatment of patients with advanced RCC or mRCC in combination with IFN-α. FDA approval came as a result of the phase III AVOREN trial. RCC patients following previous nephrectomy were randomized to receive either bevacizumab plus IFN-α or placebo plus IFN-α (Escudier et al., 2007a). The addition of bevacizumab to IFN-α significantly improved both the overall response rate (ORR) (30.6 vs. 12.4%, P<0.0001) and PFS (10.2 vs. 5.4 months). Subgroup analysis, however, indicated that the advantage in PFS related only to favourable and intermediate risk patients and not to the poor risk group. The final overall survival (OS) results reported no significant difference between the bevacizumab and control groups (23.3 vs. 21.3 months). However, these findings may have been influenced by the fact that 63% of patients in the placebo plus IFN-α group and 55% of patients in the bevacizumab plus IFN-α group received second-line therapy with other agents (Escudier et al., 2010).

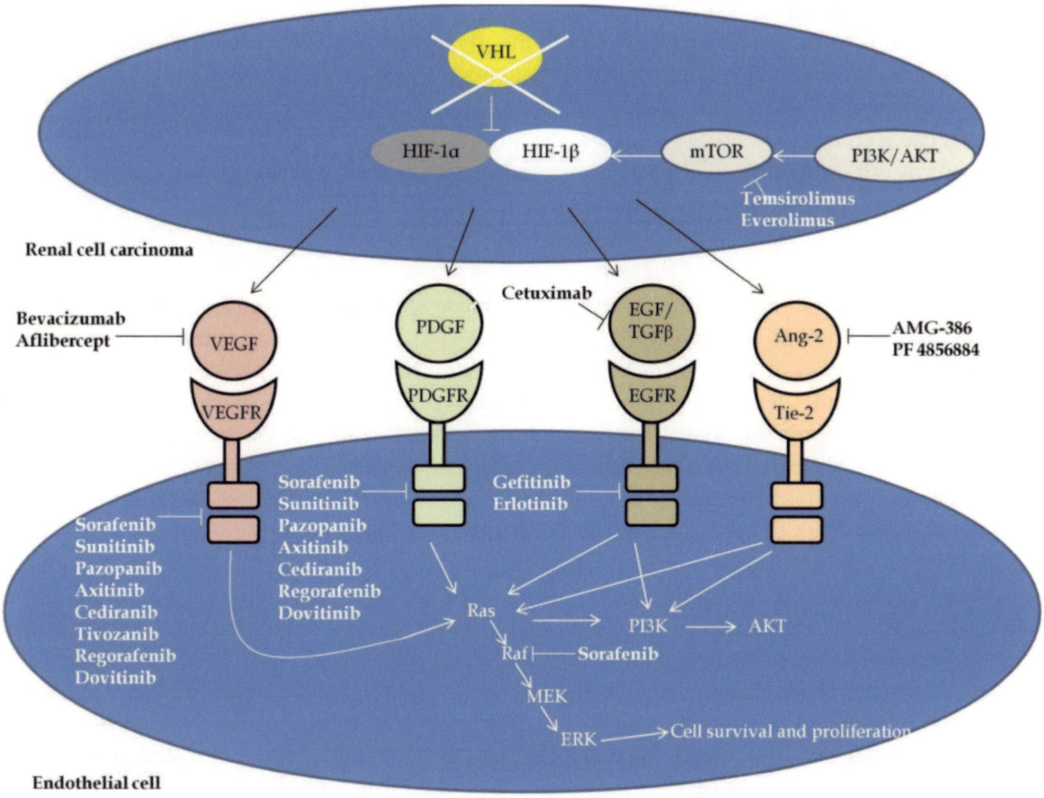

Fig. 1. Schematic representation of the signalling pathways contributing to angiogenesis and cell proliferation in RCC and the targeted agents which inhibit them. HIF activation upregulates the expression of VEGF, PDGF, EGF and Ang-2. Binding of these ligands to their receptors induces downstream activation of MAPK signalling, resulting in angiogenesis. Abbreviations; VHL: Von Hippel Lindau; HIF: hypoxia-inducible factor; mTOR: mammalian target of rapamycin; PI3K: phosphoinositol-3 kinase; VEGF(R): vascular endothelial growth factor (receptor); PDGF(R): platelet-derived growth factor (receptor); EGF(R): epidermal growth factor (receptor); TGF-β: transforming growth factor beta; Ang-2: angiopoietin 2. Inhibitory arrows (⊣) show clinically available or in development therapeutic agents for the treatment of RCC and mRCC.

2.1.2 Aflibercept

Aflibercept is an engineered fusion protein designed to interact with all isoforms of VEGF and to placental growth factor (PLGF), thereby preventing them from binding to VEGFRs. It is composed of the extracellular domain 2 of VEGFR1 and extracellular domain 3 of VEGFR2 fused to an Fc segment of human IgG1 (Wulff et al., 2002). Aflibercept appears to have a greater affinity for VEGF than bevacizumab, resulting in a more complete obstruction of VEGF signalling. This together with the fact that aflibercept binds to PLGF while bevacizumab does not, may explain why preclinical studies have shown aflibercept to be more effective than bevacizumab (Kim et al., 2002).

2.2 Receptor tyrosine kinase inhibitors (RTKIs)

The intracellular kinase activity of growth factor receptors also provides an attractive target for therapeutic intervention. Three receptor tyrosine kinase inhibitors are currently available for the treatment of clear cell RCC and many more are in development (Figure 1). By targeting the intracellular tyrosine kinase domain of multiple growth factor receptors these drugs inhibit not only the VEGF pathway but also the platelet derived growth factor (PDGF) pathway as well as other kinases critical for proliferation and angiogenesis.

2.2.1 Sorafenib

Sorafenib was the first multi-targeted kinase inhibitor approved for the treatment of patients with cytokine-refractory advanced RCC or mRCC. It is a potent small molecule dual-action inhibitor, first identified in *in vitro* assays as an inhibitor of Ras signalling. Sorafenib also inhibits VEGFRs and PDGFRs (Wilhelm et al., 2004). As multiple kinases are inhibited by sorafenib it is difficult to determine the relative contribution of each target to the anti-tumour activity of this drug. Preclinical studies in a variety of cancer models suggest sorafenib acts on both tumour cells and tumour vasculature by inhibiting cellular proliferation and angiogenesis pathways (Wilhelm et al., 2008).

Sorafenib's approval by the FDA in 2005 was as a result of a phase III trial namely; Treatment Approaches in Renal Cell Cancer Global Evaluation Trial (TARGET). All participants had advanced RCC and had experienced disease progression in spite of the then standard cytokine therapy. Patients were randomly assigned to receive sorafenib or placebo (Escudier et al., 2007b). At the first interim analysis the ORR was 10% for sorafenib compared with 2% for placebo. Also, sorafenib treated patients had a significant PFS advantage of 5.5 months versus 2.8 months for the placebo group. At this point those patients initially assigned to receive placebo were allowed to switch to sorafenib, potentially obscuring differences in end point results. In fact the final analysis of all patients registered in the trial did not show a statistically significant difference in the OS of the initial intent-to-treat population (17.8 vs. 15.2 months in sorafenib and placebo treated patients, respectively). However, a secondary analysis was performed in which patients who crossed over to sorafenib after initial treatment with placebo were censored. This demonstrated a significant benefit for sorafenib treatment with a median OS of 17.8 months compared to 14.3 months for placebo (Escudier et al., 2009). In terms of side effect profile sorafenib treated patients reported fewer adverse effects and a better overall quality of life than those receiving IFN-α. Both hypertension and skin toxicity, in general, are common manifestations of toxicity with multiple tyrosine kinase inhibitors, with incidences of 17% and 40% respectively, outlined in the TARGET trial. Other adverse effects associated with sorafenib treatment are diarrhea (Escudier et al., 2007b), and an additive loss of muscle mass above that usually observed in patients with advanced cancer (Antoun et al., 2010).

2.2.2 Sunitinib

Sunitinib is a RTKI designed to prevent cells from responding to the elevated level of pro-angiogenic signals associated with RCC. It is an orally available, small molecule, multi-targeted kinase inhibitor with activity against VEGFRs, PDGFRs, fms-like tyrosine kinase receptor-3 (FLT-3) and stem cell factor receptor (c-KIT). Sunitinib is classified as an ATP competitive inhibitor. It received accelerated approval by the FDA in 2006 based on responses in patients with mRCC who had failed cytokine therapy. Regular approval was obtained in 2007 as a result of a phase III study evaluating sunitinib as a first-line therapy compared with IFN-α. Results of the trial demonstrated a considerable advantage for sunitinib over IFN-α and both OS rates and PFS were significantly higher for the sunitinib treated group (Motzer et al., 2007a; Motzer et al., 2009). Sunitinib is now the standard of care for initial therapy of good to moderate prognosis mRCC patients. OS of over two years is a marked improvement on the one year OS rates observed before the advent of targeted kinase inhibitor therapy (Motzer et al., 2009).

As sunitinib inhibits multiple kinases and therefore blocks several signalling pathways, numerous side effects are associated with treatment. These, however, are favourable when compared to the significant toxicity profile associated with the previous therapeutic option for RCC i.e. immunotherapy. In the phase III trial which led to the approval of sunitinib, slightly different toxicity profiles were observed between the two treatment groups. Sunitinib treated patients more commonly experienced diarrhea, hypertension, hand-foot syndrome, neutropenia and thrombocytopenia while fatigue occurred more commonly in the IFN-α group. Overall, however, patients who received sunitinib reported a better quality of life compared to patients treated with IFN-α.

2.2.3 Pazopanib

Pazopanib is the latest multiple kinase inhibitor approved for the first-line treatment of patients with advanced RCC. It inhibits signalling by VEGFRs, PDGFRs, and c-KIT by competitively binding to the ATP enzymatic pocket of the RTK. Pazopanib differs from sunitinib and sorafenib as the range of targets it potently inhibits is narrower. FDA approval followed a phase III trial involving clear cell (or predominately clear cell) RCC patients with no previous treatment history (54%), or who had progressed following a single prior cytokine treatment (46%) (Sternberg et al., 2010). Patients were randomized to receive either pazopanib or placebo daily. In the overall population the primary end point of PFS was significantly higher in the pazopanib group compared to placebo (9.2 vs. 4.2 months). The ORR for the pazopanib group was 30%. Although a non-significant improvement in median OS of 22.9 months for the pazopanib group versus 20.5 months for the placebo group was reported, this analysis had been confounded by the early and high level of patient cross-over from placebo to pazopanib upon progression (Sternberg, 2010).

The toxicity profile associated with pazopanib treatment is similar to both sunitinib and sorafenib. The most common effects observed include hypertension, diarrhea, nausea, hair depigmentation and asthenia. Clinical trials cannot easily be compared, however, as evident from a phase III trial of pazopanib which demonstrated lower incidence of hand-foot syndrome, diarrhea and asthenia compared with sunitinib and sorafenib. Conversely, the incidence of hypertension associated with pazopanib treatment in the phase III trial is high (40%) when compared to sunitinib and sorafenib trials (Lang & Harrison, 2010).

2.2.4 In development

The new generation of RTKIs in development for the treatment of RCC display greater potency and selectivity for VEGFRs compared to the established kinase inhibitors discussed above. It is hoped that this increased potency and high specificity will give rise to enhanced anti-tumour activity. Furthermore, the absence of off-target (non-VEGFR) inhibition may result in less toxicity than is normally associated with kinase inhibitors in general.

2.2.5 Axitinib (AG-013736)

Axitinib is an orally available RTKI. Picomolar concentrations are sufficient for axitinib to inhibit VEGFRs, while it inhibits PDGFR-β and c-KIT at low nanomolar concentrations (Hu-Lowe et al., 2008). In this study and others (Inai et al., 2004) axitinib in mouse models has demonstrated anti-tumour, anti-angiogenic and anti-metastatic properties as well as having an ability to induce central necrosis. Axitinib is now being looked at for the second-line treatment of advanced RCC. In a phase II trial of patients with cytokine-refractory mRCC (Rixe et al., 2007), axitinib displayed an ORR of 44.2% and median PFS of 15.7 months, greater than any agent investigated for mRCC treatment to-date. However, this efficacy has not been examined in comparative trials with other targeted agents.

2.2.6 Cediranib (AZD2171)

Cediranib is an ATP-competitive inhibitor of RTKs and like axitinib is a potent inhibitor of VEGFRs and PDGFR-β at subnanomolar concentrations (Gomez-Rivera et al., 2007; Takeda et al., 2007). In a recent placebo controlled phase II trial, a median PFS of 12.1 months was observed in patients treated with cediranib compared to 2.7 months for those who received placebo. Furthermore, the mean change in tumour size in patients receiving cediranib was a 20% decrease versus a mean increase of 19% for patients randomized to placebo (Bhargava & Robinson, 2011).

2.2.7 Tivozanib (AV-951)

Tivozanib is an orally active RTKI and is selective for VEGFRs at picomolar concentrations (Nakamura et al., 2006). In a phase II trial, clear cell RCC patients who had undergone nephrectomy displayed an ORR of 32% to 1.5 mg tivozanib daily. The median PFS for patients was 14.8 months (Bhargava et al., 2010). This potency combined with the selectivity of tivozanib for VEGFRs reduces the inhibition of off-target kinases, resulting in less toxicity. The most common side effects reported in this trial were hypertension and dysphonia while incidences of other toxicities usually associated with RTKIs (fatigue, diarrhea and hand-foot syndrome) were low. The occurrence of fewer toxicities together with the specificity of tivozanib allows it to be safely combined at full dose and scheduled with another targeted agent. For example, preliminary results of a phase I trial combining tivozanib and the mTOR inhibitor temsirolimus in mRCC patients reported no dose limiting toxicities (Fishman et al., 2009).

2.2.8 Regorafenib

Regorafenib is a potentially significant multi-kinase inhibitor in that it inhibits the traditional targets of VEGFRs, PDGF-β and fibroblast growth factor (FGF)-1, as well as the endothelium specific receptor tyrosine kinase Tie-2. The inhibition of targets both within and external to the VEGF axis may offer valuable therapeutic advantages when it comes to avoiding resistance and enhancing the efficacy of targeted therapy. A phase II trial of regorafenib in mRCC patients showed that those receiving regorafenib had a 27% partial response and a 42% stable disease rate (Eisen et al., 2009).

2.2.9 Dovitinib (TKI258)

Dovitinib is also a promising agent targeting VEGFRs, PDGFRs, FLT3 as well as FGF receptors namely FGFR3. This is significant as not only does the FGF angiogenic signalling pathway provide a potential mechanism of resistance to VEGF therapy, activating mutations or upregulation of FGF/FGFRs have been identified in RCC (Emoto et al., 1994). Members of the FGF family are involved in proliferation, differentiation and migration of a range of cell types. A phase II study of dovitinib in previously treated advanced RCC or mRCC patients has reported results which include a median PFS and OS of 6.1 and 16 months, respectively (Angevin et al., 2011).

3. Targeting EGFR

Disruption of EGF signalling is a popular therapeutic mechanism in a number of cancer types. As the expression of ligands of the EGFR (including EGF and the angiogenesis promoting transforming growth factor (TGF)-β) is upregulated by *VHL* inactivation, the validity of this approach in clear cell RCC was explored in a number of trials. In single-agent EGFR inhibitor trials, gefitinib (a selective EGFR TKI) and cetuximab (a recombinant mouse-human mAb) were administered as monotherapy. Neither agent demonstrated a complete or partial response (Staehler et al., 2005). In a randomized phase II trial, clear cell RCC patients received either bevacizumab or bevacizumab plus the EGFR inhibitor erlotinib. The results showed identical median PFS and ORR between the two groups (Bukowski et al., 2007). EGFR inhibition therefore does not appear to be a viable approach for the treatment of clear cell RCC. A possible reason for this may be the rarity of EGFR mutations in RCC, when compared to other cancers (Dancey, 2004). Furthermore, the activators of EGFR signalling which are upregulated in RCC can also initiate VEGFR signalling, making the inhibition of EGFR alone insufficient to disrupt tumour proliferation and angiogenesis.

4. Targeting PDGF

Members of the PDGF family include PDGF-A, -B, -C and –D and mediate their effects through binding to PDGFR-α and –β leading to the activation of various signalling pathways giving rise to tumour growth (Guo et al., 2003; Pietras et al., 2003). High levels of PDGF-D has been shown to be associated with RCC and its progression has been linked to PDGF-D/PDGFR-β signalling and PDGFR-α expression (Sulzbacher et al., 2003). Although there is not a wealth of data published on PDGF and PDGFR in RCC there are currently many drugs either clinically available or in development that target this RTK as outlined above and in Figure 1.

5. Limitations of currently available targeted agents

Comparison of the relative benefit of each targeted treatment in advanced RCC and mRCC is exceptionally difficult. Trials conducted targeting RTKs involved varied patient populations with differences in prior treatment status, prognosis and histology of RCC. According to Flaherty & Puzanov the easiest comparison is ORR. This comparison identifies two groups: bevacizumab and sorafenib generate a response rate of ≤10%, while sunitinib and pazopanib induce a response in ≥30% of patients. However, this does not reflect any clinical benefit as higher response rates do not appear to be associated with improved PFS or OS (Flaherty & Puzanov, 2010).

Resistance is a major problem with both older and newer therapies as well as mono and poly therapies. Few complete responses are associated with any of the targeted therapies discussed. All patients will eventually develop resistance and progress, usually within 8 to 16 months (Sosman & Puzanov, 2009). A number of mechanisms have been described outlining how resistance can occur. Sorafenib, sunitinib and pazopanib therapy is associated with a significant increase in VEGF production (Deprimo et al., 2007; Kumar et al., 2007; Veronese et al., 2006). Resistance may occur if the increase in VEGF reaches a threshold that can overcome the inhibition. Another hypothesis has been examined in animal models of tumour angiogenesis. These models outline that the inhibition of VEGF or VEGFR leads to upregulation of PDGF and basic FGF (bFGF) production by tumours activating alternative pathways for angiogenic signalling (Fernando et al., 2008). Despite the overlap of targets and inevitable resistance, however, RCC tumours do not appear to be totally cross-resistant to sequential therapy with different agents. In a phase II study, patients who had progressed on sunitinib underwent treatment with sorafenib. Objective responses resulted in 10% of patients with a median PFS of 16 weeks (Di Lorenzo et al., 2009). A possible explanation is that when the initial inhibitor is removed (once resistance has occurred and the tumour has progressed), cells revert back to VEGF signalling.

Presently, it is hoped that combination therapies for the treatment of patients with RCC will see improvements in PFS, ORR and OS greater than those seen with any single agent. There are two options for the combination of targeted therapies i.e. vertical blockade and horizontal blockade. Vertical blockade involves targeting several steps along a single signalling pathway. This is an attractive option in treatment of RCC combining drugs which inhibit hypoxia-inducible factor (HIF) translation, VEGF or VEGFR. This approach could provide an opportunity to overcome the resistance associated with increased levels of VEGF. A phase I trial evaluated the potential benefit of combining sorafenib with bevacizumab in mRCC patients (Sosman, 2008). Due to toxicity, the dosage of both agents had to be reduced from their usual levels to half the recommended dose of bevacizumab and one-quarter the usual dose of sorafenib. Despite this a 50% response rate was observed, a vast improvement on the 10-15% achieved with full doses of each agent alone. The combination strategy of horizontal blockade entails simultaneously targeting more than one signalling pathway crucial for tumour cell survival and proliferation. Horizontal blockade is an appealing option as combining VEGFR inhibitors with other tyrosine kinase inhibitors may prove useful in preventing resistance by the mechanism of alternative angiogenic pathways.

6. PI3K/AKT/mTOR signalling pathway

The phosphatidylinositol 3-kinase/protein kinase B/mammalian target of rapamycin-pathway (PI3K/AKT/mTOR-pathway) is one of the most common aberrant pathways activated in cancer, regulating many known oncogenic pathways including apoptosis, proliferation and cell migration (Carracedo & Pandolfi, 2008; Klein & Levitzki, 2009; Inoki et al., 2005). Activation of PI3K occurs at the cell membrane in response to several RTKs including the EGFR, the insulin-like growth factor receptor (IGFR) and the PDGFR leading to the production of the second messenger phosphatidylinositol-3,4,5-triphosphate (PIP3). Levels of PIP3 are tightly regulated by the tumour suppressor phosphatase and tensin homolog (PTEN), serving as the negative regulator of the PI3K/AKT/mTOR pathway. AKT is recruited to the cell membrane by PIP3 and phosphorylated to its fully activated form by phosphoinositide dependent protein kinase 1 (PDK1). Activated AKT can directly activate mTOR by phosphorylation or indirectly through inactivation of the tuberous sclerosis complex 2 (TSC2) which normally inhibits mTOR (Figure 2).

mTOR is a 290kDa serine/threonine protein kinase and is highly conserved from fungi to mammals. It forms multimolecular complexes and plays a key role in diverse signalling events such as growth, proliferation, survival, angiogenesis and protein synthesis (Dowling et al., 2010). mTOR responds to a range of diverse stimuli including growth factors, cytokines, and hormones but also acts as an important sensor of cellular stresses imposed by hypoxia, pH or osmotic alterations, heat shock, oxidative stress and DNA damage. Defects in signalling components upstream of mTOR including excessive growth factor receptor activation or mutation correlates with a more aggressive tumour and a worse prognosis (Faivre et al., 2006). mTOR exists as two distinct complexes, mTOR complex 1 (mTORC1) and mTOR complex 2 (mTORC2) (Figure 2). Regulation of mTOR activation is controlled by two components of the tuberous sclerosis complex (TSC) comprising TSC1 (hamartin) and TSC2 (tuberin). When they heterodimerise mTOR is inhibited and can no longer phosphorylate downstream substrates (Dancey, 2005). Phosphorylation of TSC2 by AKT, however, promotes dissociation of the TSC1/TSC2 complex which activates the guanosine triphosphate Rheb. Rheb activity subsequently activates mTORC1. mTORC1 is bound to raptor (regulatory-associated protein of mTOR), mLST8 (mammalian lethal with sec 13 protein 8), also known as GβL and PRAS40 (proline-rich AKT substrate 40kDa) which is phosphorylated by AKT causing its dissociation from raptor and its subsequent activation. mTORC2 complexes with rictor (rapamycin-insensitive companion of mTOR), mSIN1, mLST8 and Protor-1 or Protor-2. Both complexes phosphorylate the hydrophobic motifs of AGC kinase family members. mTORC1 phosphorylates S6K and the inhibitory binding protein 4E-BP1 at Thr37 and Thr 46 which acts as a priming event essential for the phosphorylation of Ser65 and Thr70 leading to the release of eIF4E and subsequent assembly of the eIF4F complex (Gingras et al., 2001). Activation of S6K in turn leads to phosphorylation of inhibitory sites (Ser636 and 639) on the insulin receptor substrate-1 (IRS-1), thereby suppressing IRS-1 mediated activation of the PI3K/AKT pathway. mTORC2 activation leads to phosphorylation of AKT, SGK1 and PKC which control cell survival and cytoskeletal organization (Figure 2).
mTORC1 is frequently dysregulated in cancer (Guertin & Sabatini, 2007). Loss or inactivation of tumour suppressors such as p53, liver kinase B1 (LKB1), PTEN and TSC1/2 which antagonise PI3K-dependent activation of mTORC1 can promote tumourigenesis via increased signalling through mTORC1 (Sabatini, 2006; Shaw et al., 2004). Moreover, increased levels and/or phosphorylation of downstream targets of mTORC1 have been reported in various human malignancies in which they correlate with tumour aggressiveness and poor prognosis (Guertin & Sabatini, 2007; Mamane et al., 2006). Collectively these studies suggest that aberrant mTORC1 signalling is linked to dysregulated control in cancer and for this reason the spotlight has been shone on mTORC1 as a possible therapeutic target for anti-cancer therapy.

6.1 mTOR and RCC

As outlined above the signalling network controlled by the PI3K/AKT/mTOR axis is very often found to be dysregulated in human malignancy. There is a wealth of data to support the notion that signalling through mTOR is dysregulated in RCC. This makes this cancer type in particular an attractive target for mTOR inhibitor therapy. RCC demonstrates increased phosphorylation of AKT, S6K1 and mTOR as well as increased expression of PTEN and disrupted TSC complexes (Pantuck et al., 2007). mTOR activation ultimately leads to increased production of angiogenic factors leading to a highly vascularised tumour which is evident in RCC.

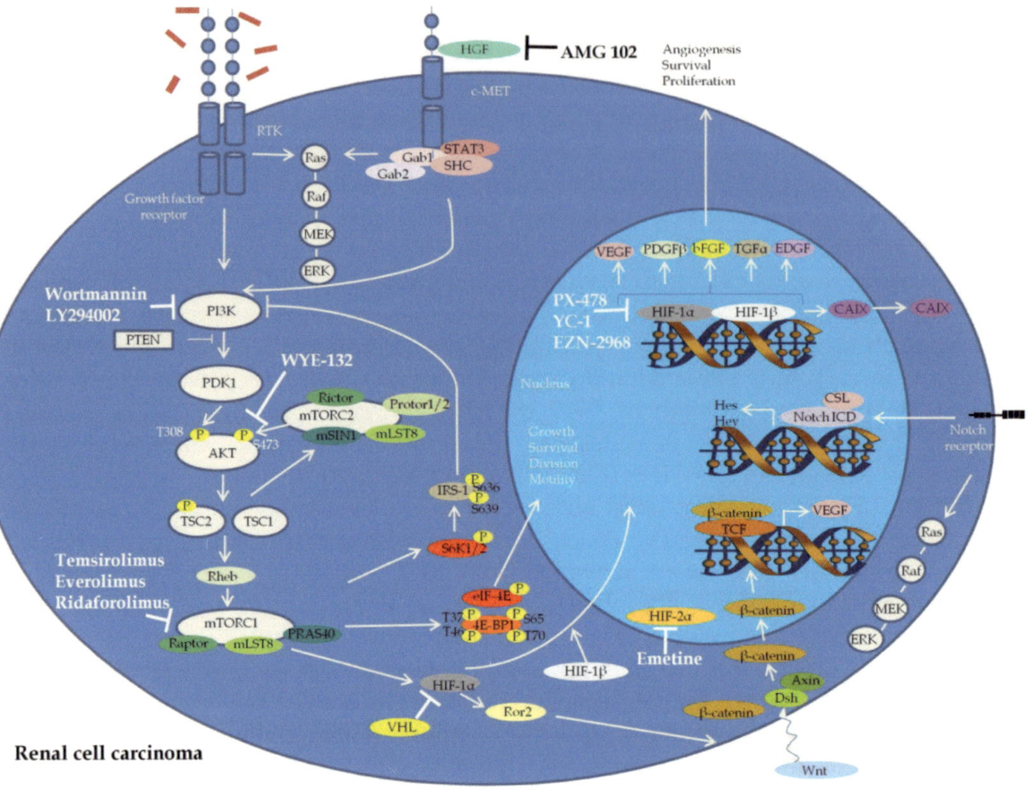

Fig. 2. Schematic representation of mTOR signalling, phosphatidylinositide 3'OH-kinase/AKT/mTOR signalling, Wnt/β-catenin signalling, HGF signalling and core NOTCH signalling pathways. In relation to growth factor signalling, PI3K activates downstream mTORC1 giving rise to HIF-1α activation, which in turn switches on gene expression required for angiogenesis and cell proliferation in endothelial cells. HGF binding to MET leads to its phosphorylation and subsequent recruitment of adapter proteins such as Gab1, Gab2, SHC, STAT3 and PI3K with downstream activation of Ras/MAPK and PI3K/AKT pathways. Wnt pathway activation leads to hypophosphorylated β-catenin where it translocates into the nucleus and forms a complex with TCF. Ligand binding to the Notch receptor leads to release of the intracellular domain (ICD) of Notch. Notch ICD subsequently translocates into the nucleus, where it forms a complex with essential cofactors such as the transcription factor CSL. This complex mediates the transcription of target genes such as HES and HEY. Abbreviations; RTK: receptor tyrosine kinase; PI3K: phosphatidylinositol 3-kinase; PDK1: phosphoinositide dependent protein kinase 1; PTEN: phosphatase and tensin homolog; mTOR: mammalian target of rapamycin; TSC: tuberous sclerosis complex; mLST8: mammalian lethal with sec 13 protein 8; PRAS40: prolin-rich AKT substrate 40 kDa; IRS-1: insulin receptor substrate-1; VHL: von Hippel-Lindau; HIF: hypoxia inducible factor; TCF; T cell factor; HGF: hepatocyte growth factor; CSL: CBF1, Suppressor of hairless, Lag-1; HES: hairy enhancer of split; Hey: hairy enhancer of split related with YRPW. Inhibitory arrows (┤) show clinically available or in development therapeutic targets for the treatment of RCC and mRCC.

mTOR inhibitors were originally developed as immunosuppressants for patients undergoing transplantation with rapamycin (also known as sirolimus or Rapamune®) being the first mTOR inhibitor identified. Clinical experience and subsequent trials identified the anti-proliferative (Schmelzle & Hall, 2000) and anti-angiogenic (Del Bufalo et al., 2006) properties of these agents in various cancer types, including RCC. This is of particular clinical importance as RCC demonstrates significant uncontrolled angiogenesis. More specifically mTORC1 activity is inhibited by rapamycin and associated analogs (temsirolimus, everolimus and ridaforolimus) which are collectively termed rapalogs. mTORC2, however, is largely insensitive to rapalogs, although prolonged treatment may be able to reduce mTORC2 activity in some cell types (Sarbassov et al., 2006).

6.1.1 mTOR inhibitors-rapamycin

Rapamycin is a naturally occurring macrolide triene antibiotic that acts as a specific, allosteric inhibitor of mTORC1 (Hay & Sonenberg, 2004). Rapamycin either associates with the immunophilin FKBP12 (FK 506-binding protein of 12 kDa) and the resulting complex interacts with the FRB (FKBP12-rapamycin binding) domain located in the C-terminus of mTOR or directly to FRB. This binding prevents the binding of mTORC1 to raptor which is thought to uncouple it from its substrates 4E-BPs and S6Ks (Oshiro et al., 2004). The ability of rapamycin to suppress both cellular proliferation and growth through its interaction with mTORC1 indicated that it could be used as an anti-cancer agent (Faivre et al., 2006). This lead to the development of rapamycin analogs (rapalogs) which display the same pharmacodynamics as the parent drug but have improved pharmacokinetic properties.

6.1.2 Temsirolimus

Temsirolimus (Torisel®), also known as CCI-779, is a macrocyclic lactone and a water-soluble ester prodrug of rapamycin. It is administered by i.v. injection, is rapidly cleared from the plasma and is converted by CYP4503A4/5 into rapamycin. It binds with high affinity to the immunophilin FKBP12 and selectively inhibits mTORC1 with no effect on mTORC2 (Le Tourneau et al., 2008). Inhibition of mTORC1 kinase activity results in decreased phosphorylation of S6K and 4E-BP1. In addition by inhibiting mTORC1 it has been shown to reduce expression of HIF-1α and -2α which leads to decreased VEGF and PDGF expression (Thomas et al., 2006). Thus, the clinical efficacy of temsirolimus reflects bimodal phamacodynamics resulting in null signalling of RTK cascades and inhibition of protein synthesis can result in inhibition of cell cycle and tumourigenesis. Temsirolimus was approved as first-line therapy for patients with mRCC in the US and Europe in May 2007 demonstrating improved efficacy in poor-prognosis patients in comparison with IFN-α (Hudes et al., 2009). The efficacy of temsirolimus in the second-line setting remains unclear. However, recently it has demonstrated disease control rate of 70% and overall median time to progression of four months in intermediate to poor-prognosis patients with VEGF-refractory mRCC (Mackenzie et al., 2011). Side effects of the drug include diarrhoea, asthenia stomatitis, rash, nausea, anorexia, hypertension, dyspnea, hyperglycaemia, hypercholesterolemia and anemia.

6.1.3 Temsirolimus plus immunotherapy combination

Temsirolimus was first investigated as combination therapy with IFN-α in phase I/II study (Motzer et al., 2007b). This study revealed that the combination of the two had an accepted safety profile and displayed anti-tumour activity in patients with mRCC. A pivotal phase III trial was also carried out comparing temsirolimus or temsirolimus plus IFN-α with IFN-α alone in patients with mRCC. In summary, the median OS time was significantly longer with temsirolimus alone than with IFN-α alone (10.9 months versus 7.3 months, respectively), and combination therapy with temsirolimus and IFN-α did not lead to a significantly longer median OS time than with IFN-α alone (8.4 months versus 7.3 months, respectively) (Hudes et al., 2007).

6.1.4 Temsirolimus plus anti-angiogenics combination

Phase I studies examining the efficacy of temsirolimus with sunitinib have not shown sufficient safety to-date. Trials using temsirolimus in combination with sunitinib and temsirolimus in combination with sorafenib were discontinued owing to significant toxicity (Patel et al., 2009). The efficacy of temsirolimus plus bevacizumab has also been studied but again based on toxicity profiles a phase II trial has indicated that this combination cannot be recommended for patients with mRCC (Negrier et al., 2011). In summary, the combined usage of temsirolimus and anti-angiogenic agents has proved disappointing to date, phase III trials are still continuing whose results may shed light on possible best practice for combination therapy in the near future.

6.2 Everolimus

Everolimus (Afinitor®) is an orally bioavailable hydroxyethyl ester of rapamycin. Like temsirolimus it is an inhibitor of mTORC1 and was approved on March 30th, 2009 for patients suffering from advanced RCC following failure when treated with previous TKI therapy (de Reijke et al., 2009). It has now become the standard second-line agent after the approved first-line drugs sunitinib and/or sorafenib (Soulieres, 2009).

6.2.1 Everolimus plus anti-angiogenics combination

The combination of everolimus and the VEGFR TKIs are showing promise in initial studies. A phase II study of everolimus plus sorafenib has been prompted following successful completion of a phase I trial with the combination of both demonstrating acceptable toxicity and evidence of anti-tumour activity in patients with previously untreated mRCC (Harzstark et al., 2011). Similarly, a phase II trial of everolimus plus sunitinib is warranted following successful maximum-tolerated dose of everolimus plus sunitinib in patients with mRCC (Kroog et al., 2009). In contrast, everolimus plus imatinib is not recommended for future studies following results from a phase II study in previously treated patients with mRCC as the combination did not demonstrate a three month PFS rate of 49%, which did not meet the specified criteria for continuation (Ryan et al., 2011). Finally, in a phase II trial with two different mRCC patient cohorts, one with and one without prior TKI treatment, everolimus plus bevacizumab was active and well tolerated (Hainsworth et al., 2010). This regimen which uses full doses of each agent, is being evaluated as first-line therapy in a phase II study, RECORD (Renal Cell Cancer Treatment With Oral RAD 001 Given Daily)-2.

6.3 Ridaforolimus

The mTOR inhibitor, ridaforolimus (formerly deforolimus), is yet another promising rapamycin analog in RCC treatment but not yet approved. Ridaforolimus (also known as AP23573), a non-prodrug of rapamycin, has demonstrated prominent anti-proliferative activity against a range of cancers (Hartford et al., 2009). The most common side effects associated with ridaforolimus to-date include stomatitis, fatigue, diarrhoea and thrombocytopenia. Important additional information such as OS and the safety profile of ridaforolimus has yet to be identified.

6.4 Combination therapy

At present there are numerous ongoing and planned studies evaluating the efficacy of both temsirolimus and everolimus with other targeted therapies including VEGF ligand competitors, VEGFR inhibitors, AKT inhibitors, p70S6R inhibitors, tubulin inhibitors, IGF-1R antagonists and Bcr-ABL antagonists (Pal & Figlin, 2011). Information pertaining to the successes associated with these exploratory trials is limited at present.

6.5 New mTOR inhibitors

Presently, temsirolimus and everolimus are approved for the treatment of mRCC. Despite their efficacy there are some drawbacks including resistance but also the fact that they are both specific mTORC1 inhibitors that lack activity against mTORC2. This allows the latter to activate AKT. Indeed, increased activation i.e. phosphorylation of AKT has been documented in tumour biopsies isolated from patients treated with rapalogs (O'Reilly et al., 2006). In addition the crosstalk with other pathways such as MEK/ERK on AKT could limit the efficacy of mTOR inhibitors. There are reports of newer drugs targeting mTORC2 as well as MAPK interacting pathways. New mTOR inhibitors are not rapalogs but are small molecule inhibitors resembling TKIs. They bind competitively and reversibly to the mTOR-ATP binding pocket blocking the enzymatic activity of the kinase. Compounds such as PP242, Torin1, WYE-354, WYE-125132 (WYE-132) and Ku-006379 suppress both mTORC1 and mTORC2 displaying more dramatic effects on cell growth, proliferation and cell cycle than rapamycin. This has been attributed to suppression of mTORC2 mediated AKT phosphorylation at Ser 473 and greater inhibition of 4E-BP1 phosphorylation (Thoreen et al., 2009). Active site mTOR inhibitors have the potential to be potent anti-cancer drugs as they inhibit mTORC2 activity which rapamycin and its analogs do not but also because they counteract the activation of AKT which can occur as a result of rapamycin-mediated disruption of the mTOR/S6K/IRS-1 negative feedback loop. To-date these potentially effective cancer therapeutic agents have yet to be investigated in patients with RCC or mRCC.

7. Targeting mTOR upstream moieties – PI3K

PI3K is a lipid kinase that converts phosphatidylinositol bisphosphate to PIP3. PI3K further recruits PDK1 and AKT to the cell membrane where PDK1 activates AKT. Because of its location upstream of mTOR, it has become another attractive target for treatment of patients with RCC to be used solely or in combination with existing mTOR inhibitors. Recently, activation of the PI3K pathway has been shown to be directly linked to adverse clinical outcomes in patients with RCC (Merseburger et al., 2008). The PI3K inhibitor prototypes wortmannin and LY294002 have been shown to decrease AKT activation and significantly reduce cell growth *in vitro* particularly in PTEN-null or PI3K-overexpressing RCCs with the latter also demonstrating *in vivo* tumour regression (Sourbier et al., 2006). Given that PI3K is highly expressed in RCC metastases, which are themselves radioresistant, newer generation PI3K inhibitors such as PX-866, with better bioavailability and less toxicity, may show utility as radiosensitizers in RCC metastases. Another chemotherapeutic drug, PI-103, has recently been shown to independently inhibit both PI3Kα and mTOR (Fan et al., 2006) thereby overcoming a potential disadvantage of rapamycin in the treatment of AKT-dependent tumors. In fact GDC-0941 which is derived from PI-103 has demonstrated improved bioavailability and partial response in breast and ovarian cancer patients. Ongoing studies using PI3K and dual PI3K/mTOR inhibitors such as SAR245408, SAR245408, NVP-BKM120 and NVP-BEZ235 modified for clinical use are ongoing (Maira et al., 2008). These have yet to be tested in patients with RCC.

7.1 PDK1

Similar to PI3K, a key mediator of AKT activation, PDK1 is poised to respond to targeted inhibition with blockade of AKT signalling (Figure 2). Both highly specific inhibitors, such as AR-12 (Arno), and inhibitors with dual function on PDK1/PI3K or PDK1/AKT are in development (Najafov et al., 2010). These targets present another potentially robust way to render the AKT pathway completely inhibited, mitigating the confounding issues of inhibition of each of the AKT family members.

7.2 AKT

AKT, also known as protein kinase B (PKB), can be activated by a number of mechanisms including PIP3 activation of PDK1 at Thr308 and at Ser473 by mTORC2 (Figure 2). Decreased expression of the inhibitory PTEN can also activate AKT (Hara et al., 2005). Upon phosphorylation (p-)AKT is known to interact with a large set of substrates, including mTOR and through inactivation of the TSC impacts many key cellular processes such as cell cycle progression and apoptosis, both of which play a vital role in oncogenesis. Recently, p-AKT expression was shown to be correlated with pathologic variables and survival, with higher levels of cytoplasmic p-AKT expression compared with nuclear p-AKT in primary RCC (Pantuck et al., 2007). Recently, a specific p-AKT (S473) inhibitor, WYE-132, has been tested on RCC cell lines and achieved complete regression of A498 large tumours when administered with bevacizumab (Yu et al., 2010).

8. Targeting downstream moieties-HIF-1α

RCC is closely linked to mutations in the von Hippel-Lindau (*VHL*) gene. A deletion of one allele of *VHL* has been identified in >90% of patients with sporadic clear cell RCC (Gnarra et al., 1994). The remaining *VHL* allele is also commonly inactivated by a deletion event or altered methylation (Nickerson et al., 2008). In normal cell conditions, the VHL protein is a direct inhibitor of the activity of a key regulator of responses to hypoxia i.e. HIF. HIFs are heterodimers and contain an α and a β subunit. VHL targets the HIF-α isoform for proteasomal degradation. This prevents it from translocating to the nucleus and binding to HIF-β which would result in the induction of over 200 target genes that contain hypoxia-response elements in their promoters. The best described of the numerous HIF targets are growth factors which promote angiogenesis and proliferation (Figures 1 and 2). Under hypoxic conditions, VHL itself is degraded. This stabilizes HIF-α within the cell and allows it to accumulate in the nucleus. Here it initiates the expression of genes which promote cell survival and growth. The effects of biallelic inactivation of the *VHL* gene in clear cell RCC cells mirror those which result from VHL degradation in response to hypoxia. Expression of HIF targets such as VEGF, PDGF, and TGF-β are upregulated.

The *VHL* gene product, pVHL, is an E3 ubiquitin ligase that promotes the proteasomal degradation of HIF-1α, -2α and -3α. Consequently, renal carcinomas with mutations in *VHL* have high steady-state levels of HIF expression. Functional studies show that HIF is sufficient for transformation caused by loss of *VHL*, thereby establishing HIF as the primary oncogenic driver in kidney cancers (Maranchie et al., 2002). mTOR increases the translation of HIF-1 and HIF-2 which in turn can drive the expression of angiogenic factors such as VEGF, PDGF-β, bFGF and TGF-α. Thus, much interest has recently focused on targeting one or both HIF factor signals for cancer therapy. EZN-2968 is an RNA antagonist that specifically binds and inhibits HIF-1α mRNA *in vitro* and *in vivo* (Greenberger et al., 2008). In this study it proved to be a potent, selective, and durable antagonist of HIF-1 mRNA and protein expression resulting in reduced prostate and glioblastoma tumor cell growth. Its efficacy in RCC has not yet been investigated. In contrast, targeting heat shock protein 90(HSP90) with 17-dimethylaminoethylamino-17-demethoxygeldanamycin (17-DMAG) which reduces levels of HIF-1α in the setting of *VHL* loss has shown promising results in clinical trials including patients with RCC (Kummar et al., 2010; Ronnen et al., 2006). Furthermore, YC-1, 3-(5'-hydroxymethyl-2'-furyl)-1-benzylindazole (an agent originally developed for circulatory disorders) and YC-1 analogs, 1, 3-disubstituted selenolo[3,2-c]pyrazole derivatives have now been found to repress HIF-1 activity and inhibit renal cancer tumour growth (Chou et al., 2010). Lastly, PX-478 (S-2-amino-3-[4'-N,N,-bis(2-chloroethyl)amino]phenyl propionic acid N-oxide dihydrochloride) an inhibitor of constitutive and hypoxia-induced HIF-1α levels and thus HIF-1 activity has proven efficacy *in vitro* with different RCC cell lines (Koh et al., 2008).

8.1 HIF-2α

HIF-2α, also referred to as endothelial PAS domain protein 1 shares 48% homology with HIF-1α. Current knowledge pertaining to the regulation of HIF-2α is somewhat lacking when compared with HIF-1α. However, the tumourigenic role of HIF-2α has been studied most extensively in RCC. Both *in vitro* and *in vivo* studies with human kidney tumours suggest that HIF-2α is more oncogenic than HIF-1α (Maranchie et al., 2002; Raval et al., 2005). RCC tumours express either HIF-1α and HIF-2α or HIF-2α alone, leaving HIF-2α expression as a common point of *VHL* mutated cancers. Moreover, consistent with this data, HIF-1α expression has been shown to decrease in advanced lesions as HIF-2α expression increases (Mandriota et al., 2002). Resulting from these observations HIF-2α is now being studied as the more important isoform for therapeutic intervention of RCC. Although several potentially important drugs targeting HIF-1α have been described (as outlined above) reports of HIF-2α are few. One potentially effective drug that needs further investigation is emetine, a protein synthesis inhibitor that blocks the translocation of peptidyl-tRNA from the acceptor site to the donor site on the riboosome. Emetine is not a novel drug (in fact it has been around for almost a century) but has been used for the treatment of bacterial, viral and amoeba *Entamoeba histolytica* infections as well as being used as an antiemetic (Zhou et al., 2005). It has been shown to induce HIF-2α downregulation in the setting of *VHL* loss in RCC cell lines. Further analysis of this drug is necessary for its efficacy in the *in vivo* setting of RCC.

9. HIF targets-Ror2

Regulated receptor tyrosine kinase-like orphan receptor 2 (Ror2) is a member of a family of orphan RTKs. Ror2 is found heavily phosphorylated in the kidney of RCC patients and is expressed highly in human RCC cell lines indicating a role for Ror2 in the pathology of RCC (Wright et al., 2009). In fact suppressed expression of Ror2 results in reduced expression of matrix metalloproteinase (MMP)-2, whose upregulation correlates with advanced stages of RCCs (Slaton et al., 2001). Thus, Ror2 represents a promising therapeutic target for patients with RCC. Although the direct target of Ror2 kinase activity has yet to be deciphered, it does appear to act as a mediator of Wnt signals in the further activation of tumour cell signalling events (Figure 2). There are currently no clinically available drugs targeting Ror2 for the treatment of RCC.

9.1 Carbonic anhydrase IX

Carbonic anhydrase IX (CAIX), a hypoxia-induced protein, is unique in that it is a cell surface protein that is present in human tumours but absent from normal tissue (Figure 2). It is found to be highly expressed in clear cell RCC and is associated with grade (Genega et al., 2010). Currently, CAIX is being pursued as a prognostic indicator, diagnostic tool and a future potential targeted therapy for the treatment of RCC. Presently, there exists a chimeric antibody (cG250) used for its localisation, but also for direct antibody-dependent cellular cytotoxicity (ADCC). Thus, it has progressed through phase 1 (Davis et al., 2007), phase 2 (Bleumer et al., 2004), and is presently undergoing a phase 3 trial (NCT00087022) in patients with RCC. In addition, cG250 accumulation in RCC lesions is extremely high and so is being investigated as a strategy to deliver tumour-sterilising radiation doses with cG250 as a carrier molecule (Divgi et al., 2004). Furthermore, preliminary research with dendritic cells loaded with CAIX-derived peptides have shown to activate the cellular and humoral immune system in patients with cytokine refractory RCC (Uemura et al., 2006). Large prospective trials, however, are required to establish dendritic cell vaccination with CAIX–derived peptides or indeed direct vaccination with these peptides.

9.2 Angiopoietins and Tie-2

Angiopoietin/Tie-2 signalling pathways are important together with VEGF/VEGFR in the process of vascular endothelial growth for angiogenesis (Figure 1). Due to the highly vascular nature of RCC identifying new anti-angiogenic agents is highly desirable in an effort to try and treat this largely refractory cancer. One such target is Tie-2, an endothelium-specific tyrosine kinase, which serves as a receptor for the family of angiopoietin ligands, angiopoietin-1 (Ang-1) and angiopoietin-2 (Ang-2), pro-angiogenic targets of HIF transcriptional activity. Binding of the former induces autophosphorylation of Tie-2, the latter antagonizes the actions of Ang-1 by competitively binding to Tie-2 without activating it. Ang-1 plays an important role in the assembly of newly formed vasculature and in the maintenance of vascular integrity. The role of Ang-2 in angiogenesis is highly dependent on the presence of other angiogenic factors, particularly VEGF. Tie-2 expression has been shown to correlate with angiopoietin-2 expression in RCC tumours (Liu et al., 2008).

Development of therapeutic drugs targeting the Angiopoietin/Tie-2 pathway differ somewhat. They may be direct inhibitors of the tyrosine kinase i.e. to target Tie-2, selective and non-selective traps to target Ang-1 or -2, or systemic delivery of angiopoietins to induce their anti-tumour effects (Huang et al., 2010). Tie-2 kinase inhibitors include CEP-11981 and CE-245677, the former is currently being evaluated in an open label phase 1 trial in patients with advanced solid tumours. The latter tested in a phase I trial has been discontinued owing to unacceptable side effects. There are currently two angiopoietin traps in clinical development. AMG-386 is an anti-angiopoietin peptibody which inhibits the interaction between ligands Ang-1 and -2 with the Tie-2 receptor. It is currently undergoing phase II trials in combination with sorafenib and sunitinib for the treatment of RCC (Huang et al., 2010). The second compound PF-4856884 (also known as CVX-060) selectively targets Ang-2 and in a phase I study demonstrated a significant reduction in RCC tumour blood flow. The mild side effect profile of both of these drugs provides an attractive basis for their combination with other anti-angiogenic or chemotherapeutic agents.

9.3 Notch

Notch signalling controls a variety of processes, involving cell fate specification, differentiation, proliferation, and survival (Artavanis-Tsakonas et al., 1999). Mammals have four Notch proteins, namely Notch 1-4, that function as receptors for five Notch ligands - Jagged1 and 2, and the delta-like ligands (DLL)-1, -3 and -4. Ligand binding leads to at least three subsequent proteolytic cleavages that release the intracellular domain (ICD) of Notch. Notch ICD subsequently translocates into the nucleus, where it forms a complex with essential cofactors such as c-promoter binding factor 1 (CBF1), mastermind-like 1 (MAML1) and the transcription factor CSL. This complex mediates the transcription of target genes such as that encoding Deltex, genes in the hairy enhancer of split (HES) and HES-related families of basic helix-loop-helix transcription factors, and others (Figure 2). Aberrant signalling within this pathway has previously been reported in multiple malignancies (Miele et al., 2006) including RCC with elevated Notch 1, 3 and Jagged-1 mRNAs (Rae et al., 2000; Sjolund et al., 2008). Elevated expression of DLL-4 has also been reported in RCCs with reduction of such basal expression having considerable effects on endothelial function important in tumour angiogenesis (Patel et al., 2005). Interestingly, Notch signalling can lead to either tumour progression or suppression depending on the cellular context (Nicolas et al., 2003, Xia et al., 2001). However, in the context of RCC, Notch signalling inhibition has lead to inhibition of RCC growth thus indicating a potential novel therapeutic pathway in RCC. Presently, there is strong evidence for signalling crosstalk between Notch and HIF-1α. Cleaved Notch ICD and HIF-1α appear to play an important point between the two signalling cascades (Gustafsson et al., 2005). Moreover, there is recent evidence to support Notch signalling linking AKT and hypoxia in melanomas (Bedogni et al., 2008). Whether this interaction is pertinent to RCC has yet to be investigated. Inhibition of Notch signalling as a strategy for cancer treatment has been proposed in numerous studies (Nickoloff et al., 2003). Two approaches have been identified; selective strategies involving antisense, mAbs and RNA interference; nonselective strategies involving soluble or cell-associated Notch decoys, γ-secretase inhibitors, intracellular MAML1 decoys and Ras signalling inhibitors (Miele et al., 2006). Currently it is too early to evaluate the true efficacy of these strategies and of the different drugs involved but what is known from present findings is that Notch inhibition in cancer deserves a thorough investigation including in patients with RCC.

9.4 Wnt/β-catenin signalling

Wnts are a family of secreted glycoproteins that regulate a wide range of cellular functions such as growth, differentiation, migration and polarity (Moon et al., 2004). Wnt signalling is controlled by the transcriptional coactivator β-catenin, which is emerging as a key molecule in the pathogenesis of renal cancer. In normal quiescent cells, β-catenin is bound to casein kinase 1, glycogen synthase kinase 3β (GSK3), adenomatosis polyposis coli protein and axin. This complex controls β-catenin phosphorylation targeting it for proteosomal degradation.

Wnt positively regulates β-catenin, preventing its phosphorylation, ubiquitination and degradation. Thus, upon Wnt pathway activation hypophosphorylated β-catenin translocates into the nucleus and forms a complex with the DNA binding protein T cell factor (TCF) (Figure 2). The β-catenin/TCF complex activates transcription of a wide range of genes including growth promoting genes such as VEGF (Easwaran et al., 2003) as well as the *MYC* oncogene which shows copy number amplification in RCC (Beroukhim et al., 2009). Wnt can also mediate its effect on cell growth and tumour promotion by activating the mTOR pathway (Inoki et al., 2006). TSC2 is phosphorylated by GSK3 for its activation and subsequent inhibition of mTOR. Wnt activates mTOR pathway by inhibiting GSK3. There are several papers outlining the involvement of Wnt signalling in RCC. Overexpression of β-catenin can induce renal tumours in mice (Sansom et al., 2005). In some RCC tumours the *APC* gene promoter is aberrantly hypermethylated providing a mechanism by which β-catenin is liberated (Battagli et al., 2003). β-catenin is also degraded by the E3-ubiquitin ligase activity of VHL and so loss of VHL in RCC has been shown to enable HGF-driven oncogenic β-catenin signalling (Peruzzi et al., 2006). In a recent article further evidence for the activation of Wnt signalling in RCC was outlined when a deletion of *CXXC4* a gene coding for Idax, an inhibitor of this pathway, was identified in aggressive RCC (Kojima et al., 2009). In addition, various Wnt antagonists such as secreted-Frizzled receptor proteins, Dickkopf 2 and Wnt inhibitory factor 1 were found to be hypermethylated and thus silenced in RCC (Awakura et al., 2008; Hirata et al., 2009; Kawakami et al., 2009). It is also possible that loss of *VHL* could lead to the combined de-repression of HIFs and β-catenin which could also lead to RCC (Linehan et al., 2009). Finally, Jade-1 (gene for apoptosis and differentiation in epithelia) has been identified as a *VHL*-interacting protein which brings about β-catenin degradation. Thus, Jade-1 is thought to function as a renal tumour suppressor (Chitalia et al., 2008). Loss of *VHL* can bring about a reduction in Jade-1 levels with subsequent increases in β-catenin levels, providing another caveat by which loss of *VHL* can promote renal tumourigenesis. In summary Wnt signalling has a dual role in the pathogenesis of RCC. It induces transcription through activation of β-catenin but also activates mTOR signalling driving cellular growth. Thus, Wnt signalling and β-catenin provide attractive targets for therapeutic intervention in RCC. At present there are no clinically available drugs targeting this pathway in RCC but may become available in the near future.

10. HGF/MET signalling

Kidney tissue is an abundant source of hepatocyte growth factor (HGF) a stromal cell-derived cytokine involved in cell proliferation, tissue regeneration, tumour growth and tumour invasion through the HGF/scatter factor (SF):c-MET pathway (Cantley et al., 1994). HGF binding to MET leads to its phosphorylation and subsequent recruitment of adapter proteins such as Gab1, Gab2, SHC, STAT3 and PI3K with downstream activation of Ras/MAPK and PI3K/AKT pathways (Figure 2) resulting in RCC growth and metastasis (Eder et al., 2009). Different studies have shown that HGF and its receptor c-MET are overexpressed in RCC and play a significant role in the progression of RCC (Horie et al., 1999; Natali et al., 1996). Moreover, *VHL*-negative RCC cells exhibit cell invasion and branching morphogenesis in response to HGF (Koochekpour et al., 1999). c-MET has also been shown to be constitutively phosphorylated in RCC and high levels of serum HGF/SF in RCC patients are associated with reduced survival (Tanimoto et al., 2008). Presently, MET is being targeted in clinical trials for the treatment of RCC (Giubellino et al., 2009). Strategies involve preventing c-MET autophosphorylation; prevention of HGF binding to c-MET and lastly targeting the signalling cascade of activated c-MET (Toschi & Janne, 2008). One such investigational drug is AMG 102, a fully human mAb that blocks HGF/SF binding to c-EMT and blocks signalling events driving tumour proliferation, migration, invasion and survival (Figure 2). Reports of a phase II trial with AMG 102 identified that although the drug brought about tumour burden reduction and long-term disease stability, it was unclear from the study whether this drug is capable of tumour growth inhibition in a histologically diverse population of patients with mRCC (Schoffski et al., 2010). Other drugs currently in development include foretinib (GSK1363089) an oral multi kinase inhibitor of MET and VEGFRs (Kataoka et al., 2011), ARQ 197, a selective non-ATP competitive inhibitor of MET (Adjei et al., 2011) and a range of orally available c-MET kinase inhibitors namely (R)-3-[1-(2,6-dichloro-3-fluoro-phenyl)-ethoxy]-5-(1-piperidin-4-yl-1H-pyrazol-4-yl)-pyridin-2-ylamine (PF02341066) and 2-[4-(3-quinolin-6-ylmethyl-3H-[1,2,3]triazolo[4,5-b]pyrazin-5-yl)-pyrazol-1-yl]-ethanol (PF04217903) (Yamazaki et al., 2011). The efficacy of these drugs have yet to be investigated in patients with RCC. Thus, further investigations of these potentially effective therapeutic drugs is warranted at this time.

11. Conclusions and future directions

RCC is similar to other cancer types in that it is asymptomatic initially with a lack of early warning signs. This results in a high percentage of patients presenting with metastasis at diagnosis or indeed relapse following nephrectomy. RCC is also known for its unpredictable clinical behaviour. Historically RCC and mRCC has been associated with treatment resistance and poor prognosis. However, with ever increasing knowledge of angiogenesis and aberrant signalling pathways in patients with RCC recent basic and clinical developments has exerted a substantial impact on outcomes for patients with mRCC.

Throughout the past fifteen years there has been an increased understanding of the tumour biology of RCC. There is now a myriad of treatment options available making the treatment of RCC and mRCC immensely complex. Sequential therapy with targeted agents is currently the standard of care while combination therapies are still under active investigation. Combination therapies can provide additive or synergistic effects resulting from more complete blockade of the many aberrant signalling cascades outlined above. This approach can also prevent or delay the development of resistance that would eventually arise with single-agent therapy owing to signalling pathway redundancy. Despite recent advancements, however, current chemotherapeutics can only increase the overall survival of patients from weeks to months and unfortunately cannot cure RCC. Combination regimes have many drawbacks and in many instances have not proven beneficial in terms of inferior efficacy and excessive toxicity. It is also clear from the multitude of described and ongoing clinical trials that patient response to targeted agents is not universal. Thus, we have reached the stage where there is compelling need to identify new combinations with the goal of providing maximal efficacy with manageable toxicity. Increased knowledge of mechanisms of disease, drug resistance, new targets and new targeted agents may eventually provide optimal strategies for patients with RCC and mRCC.

Another area of note to improve the treatment of patients with RCC and mRCC is the identification of genetic and epigenetic markers as promising biomarkers (Pal et al., 2010; Vickers & Heng 2010) . This may indicate the suitability of a patient to treatment with one agent above another and also the optimal sequential or combination of therapies. Many RCC biomarkers have been examined over the past decade and include *VHL* gene mutation, plasma VEGF, tissue and plasma VEGFRs, tissue HIF and tissue and serum CAIX as outlined already in this report. Others include B7-H1 a cell surface glycoprotein that acts as a negative regulator of anti-tumoural T cell-mediated immunity and whose high levels of expression in patients with RCC has been associated with shorter survival (Vickers & Heng, 2010). Another prognostic biomarker includes neutrophil gelatinase-associated lipocalin (NGAL). NGAL is elevated in a number of cancers and has been linked to MMP-9, which is involved in the degradation of the extracellular matrix and therefore invasion and metastasis. Thus, lower levels of NGAL is associated with longer PFS in RCC patients (Vickers & Heng, 2010). Despite growing research in this area, however, there are currently no biomarkers used in the clinical management of patients with RCC. Future studies such as the NIH funded Cancer Genome Atlas project may provide further insight into the genome, mRNA and micro RNA transcriptome and methylome of RCC revealing the pathways and networking that is aberrant in RCC and thus aid in the identification of new biomarkers and therapeutic agents. Furthermore, the use of increasingly sophisticated integrative multivariate models which incorporate both molecular and genetic information will ultimately aid in the development of curative, non-toxic personalised therapies. Thus, research is ongoing and newer improved technologies hold promise in the expansion of our knowledge of pathogenesis and determinants of outcome. In summary, in the future researchers and clinicians alike will have to unite and develop a workable cohesive strategy to optimise use of available agents as well as those undergoing clinical trials and identify optimal strategies for the successful treatment of patients with RCC.

12. References

Adjei, A. A., Schwartz, B. & Garmey, E. (2011). Early Clinical Development of ARQ 197, a Selective, Non-ATP-Competitive Inhibitor Targeting MET Tyrosine Kinase for the Treatment of Advanced Cancers. *Oncologist,* ISSN 1549-490X (Electronic)

Angevin, E., Grünwald, V., Ravaud, A., Castellano, D. E., Lin, C., Gschwend, J. E., Harzstark, A. L., Chang, J., Wang, Y., Shi, M. M., Escudier, B. J. (2011). A phase II study of dovitinib (TKI258), an FGFR- and VEGFR-inhibitor, in patients with advanced or metastatic renal cell cancer (mRCC). *J Clin Oncol,* Vol. 29, suppl; abstr 4551,

Antoun, S., Birdsell, L., Sawyer, M. B., Venner, P., Escudier, B. & Baracos, V. E. (2010). Association of skeletal muscle wasting with treatment with sorafenib in patients with advanced renal cell carcinoma: results from a placebo-controlled study. *J Clin Oncol,* Vol. 28, No. 6, pp. 1054-1060, ISSN 1527-7755 (Electronic)

Artavanis-Tsakonas, S., Rand, M. D. & Lake, R. J. (1999). Notch signaling: cell fate control and signal integration in development. *Science,* Vol. 284, No. 5415, pp. 770-776, ISSN 0036-8075 (Print)

Awakura, Y., Nakamura, E., Ito, N., Kamoto, T. & Ogawa, O. (2008). Methylation-associated silencing of SFRP1 in renal cell carcinoma. *Oncol Rep,* Vol. 20, No. 5, pp. 1257-1263, ISSN 1021-335X (Print)

Battagli, C., Uzzo, R. G., Dulaimi, E., Ibanez de Caceres, I., Krassenstein, R., Al-Saleem, T., Greenberg, R. E. & Cairns, P. (2003). Promoter hypermethylation of tumor suppressor genes in urine from kidney cancer patients. *Cancer Res,* Vol. 63, No. 24, pp. 8695-8699, ISSN 0008-5472 (Print)

Bedogni, B., Warneke, J. A., Nickoloff, B. J., Giaccia, A. J. & Powell, M. B. (2008). Notch1 is an effector of Akt and hypoxia in melanoma development. *J Clin Invest,* Vol. 118, No. 11, pp. 3660-3670, ISSN 0021-9738 (Print)

Beroukhim, R., Brunet, J. P., Di Napoli, A., Mertz, K. D., Seeley, A., Pires, M. M., Linhart, D., Worrell, R. A., Moch, H., Rubin, M. A., Sellers, W. R., Meyerson, M., Linehan, W. M., Kaelin, W. G., Jr. & Signoretti, S. (2009). Patterns of gene expression and copy-number alterations in von-hippel lindau disease-associated and sporadic clear cell carcinoma of the kidney. *Cancer Res,* Vol. 69, No. 11, pp. 4674-4681, ISSN 1538-7445 (Electronic)

Bhargava, P., Esteves, B., Al-Adhami, M., Nosov, D., Lipatov, O. N., Lyulko, A. A., Anischenko, A. A., Chacko, R. T., Doval, D. & Slichenmyer, W. J. (2010). Activity of tivozanib (AV-951) in patients with renal cell carcinoma (RCC): Subgroup analysis from a phase II randomized discontinuation trial (RDT). *ASCO Meeting Abstracts,* Vol. 28, No. 15_suppl, pp. 4599

Bhargava, P. & Robinson, M. O. (2011). Development of second-generation VEGFR tyrosine kinase inhibitors: current status. *Curr Oncol Rep,* Vol. 13, No. 2, pp. 103-111, ISSN 1534-6269 (Electronic)

Bleumer, I., Knuth, A., Oosterwijk, E., Hofmann, R., Varga, Z., Lamers, C., Kruit, W., Melchior, S., Mala, C., Ullrich, S., De Mulder, P., Mulders, P. F. & Beck, J. (2004). A phase II trial of chimeric monoclonal antibody G250 for advanced renal cell carcinoma patients. *Br J Cancer,* Vol. 90, No. 5, pp. 985-990, ISSN 0007-0920 (Print)

Bukowski, R. M., Kabbinavar, F. F., Figlin, R. A., Flaherty, K., Srinivas, S., Vaishampayan, U., Drabkin, H. A., Dutcher, J., Ryba, S., Xia, Q., Scappaticci, F. A. & McDermott, D. (2007). Randomized phase II study of erlotinib combined with bevacizumab compared with bevacizumab alone in metastatic renal cell cancer. *J Clin Oncol,* Vol. 25, No. 29, pp. 4536-4541, ISSN 1527-7755 (Electronic)

Cantley, L. G., Barros, E. J., Gandhi, M., Rauchman, M. & Nigam, S. K. (1994). Regulation of mitogenesis, motogenesis, and tubulogenesis by hepatocyte growth factor in renal collecting duct cells. *Am J Physiol,* Vol. 267, No. 2 Pt 2, pp. F271-280, 0002-9513 (Print)

Carracedo, A. & Pandolfi, P. P. (2008). The PTEN-PI3K pathway: of feedbacks and cross-talks. *Oncogene,* Vol. 27, No. 41, pp. 5527-5541, ISSN 1476-5594 (Electronic)

Casanovas, O., Hicklin, D. J., Bergers, G. & Hanahan, D. (2005). Drug resistance by evasion of antiangiogenic targeting of VEGF signaling in late-stage pancreatic islet tumors. *Cancer Cell,* Vol. 8, No. 4, pp. 299-309, 1535-6108 (Print)

Chitalia, V. C., Foy, R. L., Bachschmid, M. M., Zeng, L., Panchenko, M. V., Zhou, M. I., Bharti, A., Seldin, D. C., Lecker, S. H., Dominguez, I. & Cohen, H. T. (2008). Jade-1 inhibits Wnt signalling by ubiquitylating beta-catenin and mediates Wnt pathway inhibition by pVHL. *Nat Cell Biol,* Vol. 10, No. 10, pp. 1208-1216, ISSN 1476-4679 (Electronic)

Chou, L. C., Huang, L. J., Hsu, M. H., Fang, M. C., Yang, J. S., Zhuang, S. H., Lin, H. Y., Lee, F. Y., Teng, C. M. & Kuo, S. C. (2010). Synthesis of 1-benzyl-3-(5-hydroxymethyl-2-furyl)selenolo[3,2-c]pyrazole derivatives as new anticancer agents. *Eur J Med Chem,* Vol. 45, No. 4, pp. 1395-1402, ISSN 1768-3254 (Electronic)

Couillard, D. R. & deVere White, R. W. (1993). Surgery of renal cell carcinoma. *Urol Clin North Am,* Vol. 20, No. 2, pp. 263-275, ISSN 0094-0143 (Print)

Dancey, J. E. (2004). Epidermal growth factor receptor and epidermal growth factor receptor therapies in renal cell carcinoma: do we need a better mouse trap? *J Clin Oncol,* Vol. 22, No. 15, pp. 2975-2977, ISSN 0732-183X (Print)

Dancey, J. E. (2005). Inhibitors of the mammalian target of rapamycin. *Expert Opin Investig Drugs,* Vol. 14, No. 3, pp. 313-328, ISSN 1744-7658 (Electronic)

Davis, I. D., Liu, Z., Saunders, W., Lee, F. T., Spirkoska, V., Hopkins, W., Smyth, F. E., Chong, G., Papenfuss, A. T., Chappell, B., Poon, A., Saunder, T. H., Hoffman, E. W., Old, L. J. & Scott, A. M. (2007). A pilot study of monoclonal antibody cG250 and low dose subcutaneous IL-2 in patients with advanced renal cell carcinoma. *Cancer Immun,* Vol. 7, No. pp. 14, ISSN 1424-9634 (Electronic)

de Reijke, T. M., Bellmunt, J., van Poppel, H., Marreaud, S. & Aapro, M. (2009). EORTC-GU group expert opinion on metastatic renal cell cancer. *Eur J Cancer,* Vol. 45, No. 5, pp. 765-773, ISSN 1879-0852 (Electronic)

Del Bufalo, D., Ciuffreda, L., Trisciuoglio, D., Desideri, M., Cognetti, F., Zupi, G. & Milella, M. (2006). Antiangiogenic potential of the Mammalian target of rapamycin inhibitor temsirolimus. *Cancer Res,* Vol. 66, No. 11, pp. 5549-5554, ISSN 0008-5472 (Print)

Deprimo, S. E., Bello, C. L., Smeraglia, J., Baum, C. M., Spinella, D., Rini, B. I., Michaelson, M. D. & Motzer, R. J. (2007). Circulating protein biomarkers of pharmacodynamic activity of sunitinib in patients with metastatic renal cell carcinoma: modulation of VEGF and VEGF-related proteins. *J Transl Med,* Vol. 5, No. pp. 32, ISSN 1479-5876 (Electronic)

Di Lorenzo, G., Carteni, G., Autorino, R., Bruni, G., Tudini, M., Rizzo, M., Aieta, M., Gonnella, A., Rescigno, P., Perdona, S., Giannarini, G., Pignata, S., Longo, N., Palmieri, G., Imbimbo, C., De Laurentiis, M., Mirone, V., Ficorella, C. & De Placido, S. (2009). Phase II study of sorafenib in patients with sunitinib-refractory metastatic renal cell cancer. *J Clin Oncol,* Vol. 27, No. 27, pp. 4469-4474, ISSN 1527-7755 (Electronic)

Divgi, C. R., O'Donoghue, J. A., Welt, S., O'Neel, J., Finn, R., Motzer, R. J., Jungbluth, A., Hoffman, E., Ritter, G., Larson, S. M. & Old, L. J. (2004). Phase I clinical trial with fractionated radioimmunotherapy using 131I-labeled chimeric G250 in metastatic renal cancer. *J Nucl Med,* Vol. 45, No. 8, pp. 1412-1421, ISSN 0161-5505 (Print)

Dowling, R. J., Topisirovic, I., Fonseca, B. D. & Sonenberg, N. (2010). Dissecting the role of mTOR: lessons from mTOR inhibitors. *Biochim Biophys Acta,* Vol. 1804, No. 3, pp. 433-439, ISSN 0006-3002 (Print)

Easwaran, V., Lee, S. H., Inge, L., Guo, L., Goldbeck, C., Garrett, E., Wiesmann, M., Garcia, P. D., Fuller, J. H., Chan, V., Randazzo, F., Gundel, R., Warren, R. S., Escobedo, J., Aukerman, S. L., Taylor, R. N. & Fantl, W. J. (2003). beta-Catenin regulates vascular endothelial growth factor expression in colon cancer. *Cancer Res,* Vol. 63, No. 12, pp. 3145-3153,ISSN 0008-5472 (Print)

Eder, J. P., Vande Woude, G. F., Boerner, S. A. & LoRusso, P. M. (2009). Novel therapeutic inhibitors of the c-Met signaling pathway in cancer. *Clin Cancer Res,* Vol. 15, No. 7, pp. 2207-2214, ISSN 1078-0432 (Print)

Eisen, T., Joensuu, H., Nathan, P., Harper, P., Wojtukiewicz, M., Nicholson, S., Bahl, A., Tomczak, P., Wagner, A. & Quinn, D. (2009). Phase II study of BAY 73-4506, a multikinase inhibitor, in previously untreated patients with metastatic or unresectable renal cell cancer. *ASCO Meeting Abstracts,* Vol. 27, No. 15S, pp. 5033

Ellis, L. M. & Hicklin, D. J. (2008). VEGF-targeted therapy: mechanisms of anti-tumour activity. *Nat Rev Cancer,* Vol. 8, No. 8, pp. 579-591, ISSN 1474-1768 (Electronic)

Emoto, N., Isozaki, O., Ohmura, E., Ito, F., Tsushima, T., Shizume, K., Demura, H. & Toma, H. (1994). Basic fibroblast growth factor (FGF-2) in renal cell carcinoma, which is indistinguishable from that in normal kidney, is involved in renal cell carcinoma growth. *J Urol,* Vol. 152, No. 5 Pt 1, pp. 1626-1631, ISSN 0022-5347 (Print)

Escudier, B., Bellmunt, J., Negrier, S., Bajetta, E., Melichar, B., Bracarda, S., Ravaud, A., Golding, S., Jethwa, S. & Sneller, V. (2010). Phase III trial of bevacizumab plus interferon alfa-2a in patients with metastatic renal cell carcinoma (AVOREN): final analysis of overall survival. *J Clin Oncol,* Vol. 28, No. 13, pp. 2144-2150, ISSN 1527-7755 (Electronic)

Escudier, B., Eisen, T., Stadler, W. M., Szczylik, C., Oudard, S., Siebels, M., Negrier, S., Chevreau, C., Solska, E., Desai, A. A., Rolland, F., Demkow, T., Hutson, T. E., Gore, M., Freeman, S., Schwartz, B., Shan, M., Simantov, R. & Bukowski, R. M. (2007b). Sorafenib in advanced clear-cell renal-cell carcinoma. *N Engl J Med,* Vol. 356, No. 2, pp. 125-134, ISSN 1533-4406 (Electronic)

Escudier, B., Eisen, T., Stadler, W. M., Szczylik, C., Oudard, S., Staehler, M., Negrier, S., Chevreau, C., Desai, A. A., Rolland, F., Demkow, T., Hutson, T. E., Gore, M., Anderson, S., Hofilena, G., Shan, M., Pena, C., Lathia, C. & Bukowski, R. M. (2009). Sorafenib for treatment of renal cell carcinoma: Final efficacy and safety results of the phase III treatment approaches in renal cancer global evaluation trial. *J Clin Oncol,* Vol. 27, No. 20, pp. 3312-3318, ISSN 1527-7755 (Electronic)

Escudier, B., Pluzanska, A., Koralewski, P., Ravaud, A., Bracarda, S., Szczylik, C., Chevreau, C., Filipek, M., Melichar, B., Bajetta, E., Gorbunova, V., Bay, J. O., Bodrogi, I., Jagiello-Gruszfeld, A. & Moore, N. (2007a). Bevacizumab plus interferon alfa-2a for treatment of metastatic renal cell carcinoma: a randomised, double-blind phase III trial. *Lancet,* Vol. 370, No. 9605, pp. 2103-2111, ISSN 1474-547X (Electronic)

Faivre, S., Kroemer, G. & Raymond, E. (2006). Current development of mTOR inhibitors as anticancer agents. *Nat Rev Drug Discov,* Vol. 5, No. 8, pp. 671-688, ISSN 1474-1776 (Print)

Fan, Q. W., Knight, Z. A., Goldenberg, D. D., Yu, W., Mostov, K. E., Stokoe, D., Shokat, K. M. & Weiss, W. A. (2006). A dual PI3 kinase/mTOR inhibitor reveals emergent efficacy in glioma. *Cancer Cell,* Vol. 9, No. 5, pp. 341-349, ISSN 1535-6108 (Print)

Fernando, N. T., Koch, M., Rothrock, C., Gollogly, L. K., D'Amore, P. A., Ryeom, S. & Yoon, S. S. (2008). Tumor escape from endogenous, extracellular matrix-associated angiogenesis inhibitors by up-regulation of multiple proangiogenic factors. *Clin Cancer Res,* Vol. 14, No. 5, pp. 1529-1539, ISSN 1078-0432 (Print)

Fishman, M. N., Srinivas, S., Hauke, R. J., Amato, R. J., Esteves, B., Dhillon, R., Cotreau, M., Al-Adhami, M., Bhargava, P. & Kabbinavar, F. F. (2009). Abstract B60: Combination of tivozanib (AV-951) and temsirolimus in patients with renal cell carcinoma (RCC): Preliminary results from a phase 1 trial. *Molecular Cancer Therapeutics,* Vol. 8, Supplement 1, pp. B60

Flaherty, K. T. & Puzanov, I. (2010). Building on a foundation of VEGF and mTOR targeted agents in renal cell carcinoma. *Biochem Pharmacol,* Vol. 80, No. 5, pp. 638-646, ISSN 1873-2968 (Electronic)

Genega, E. M., Ghebremichael, M., Najarian, R., Fu, Y., Wang, Y., Argani, P., Grisanzio, C. & Signoretti, S. (2010). Carbonic anhydrase IX expression in renal neoplasms: correlation with tumor type and grade. *Am J Clin Pathol,* Vol. 134, No. 6, pp. 873-879, ISSN 1943-7722 (Electronic)

Gingras, A. C., Raught, B., Gygi, S. P., Niedzwiecka, A., Miron, M., Burley, S. K., Polakiewicz, R. D., Wyslouch-Cieszynska, A., Aebersold, R. & Sonenberg, N. (2001). Hierarchical phosphorylation of the translation inhibitor 4E-BP1. *Genes Dev,* Vol. 15, No. 21, pp. 2852-2864, ISSN 0890-9369 (Print)

Giubellino, A., Linehan, W. M. & Bottaro, D. P. (2009). Targeting the Met signaling pathway in renal cancer. *Expert Rev Anticancer Ther,* Vol. 9, No. 6, pp. 785-793, ISSN 1744-8328 (Electronic)

Gnarra, J. R., Tory, K., Weng, Y., Schmidt, L., Wei, M. H., Li, H., Latif, F., Liu, S., Chen, F., Duh, F. M. & et al. (1994). Mutations of the VHL tumour suppressor gene in renal carcinoma. *Nat Genet,* Vol. 7, No. 1, pp. 85-90, ISSN 1061-4036 (Print)

Gomez-Rivera, F., Santillan-Gomez, A. A., Younes, M. N., Kim, S., Fooshee, D., Zhao, M., Jasser, S. A. & Myers, J. N. (2007). The tyrosine kinase inhibitor, AZD2171, inhibits vascular endothelial growth factor receptor signaling and growth of anaplastic thyroid cancer in an orthotopic nude mouse model. *Clin Cancer Res,* Vol. 13, No. 15 Pt 1, pp. 4519-4527, ISSN 1078-0432 (Print)

Gordan, J. D., Lal, P., Dondeti, V. R., Letrero, R., Parekh, K. N., Oquendo, C. E., Greenberg, R. A., Flaherty, K. T., Rathmell, W. K., Keith, B., Simon, M. C. & Nathanson, K. L. (2008). HIF-alpha effects on c-Myc distinguish two subtypes of sporadic VHL-deficient clear cell renal carcinoma. *Cancer Cell,* Vol. 14, No. 6, pp. 435-446, ISSN 1878-3686 (Electronic)

Greenberger, L. M., Horak, I. D., Filpula, D., Sapra, P., Westergaard, M., Frydenlund, H. F., Albaek, C., Schroder, H. & Orum, H. (2008). A RNA antagonist of hypoxia-inducible factor-1alpha, EZN-2968, inhibits tumor cell growth. *Mol Cancer Ther,* Vol. 7, No. 11, pp. 3598-3608, ISSN 1535-7163 (Print)

Guertin, D. A. & Sabatini, D. M. (2007). Defining the role of mTOR in cancer. *Cancer Cell,* Vol. 12, No. 1, pp. 9-22, ISSN 1535-6108 (Print)

Guo, P., Hu, B., Gu, W., Xu, L., Wang, D., Huang, H. J., Cavenee, W. K. & Cheng, S. Y. (2003). Platelet-derived growth factor-B enhances glioma angiogenesis by stimulating vascular endothelial growth factor expression in tumor endothelia and by promoting pericyte recruitment. *Am J Pathol,* Vol. 162, No. 4, pp. 1083-1093, ISSN 0002-9440 (Print)

Gustafsson, M. V., Zheng, X., Pereira, T., Gradin, K., Jin, S., Lundkvist, J., Ruas, J. L., Poellinger, L., Lendahl, U. & Bondesson, M. (2005). Hypoxia requires notch signaling to maintain the undifferentiated cell state. *Dev Cell,* Vol. 9, No. 5, pp. 617-628, ISSN 1534-5807 (Print)

Hainsworth, J. D., Spigel, D. R., Burris, H. A., 3rd, Waterhouse, D., Clark, B. L. & Whorf, R. (2010). Phase II trial of bevacizumab and everolimus in patients with advanced renal cell carcinoma. *J Clin Oncol,* Vol. 28, No. 13, pp. 2131-2136, ISSN 1527-7755 (Electronic)

Hara, S., Oya, M., Mizuno, R., Horiguchi, A., Marumo, K. & Murai, M. (2005). Akt activation in renal cell carcinoma: contribution of a decreased PTEN expression and the induction of apoptosis by an Akt inhibitor. *Ann Oncol,* Vol. 16, No. 6, pp. 928-933, ISSN 0923-7534 (Print)

Hartford, C. M., Desai, A. A., Janisch, L., Karrison, T., Rivera, V. M., Berk, L., Loewy, J. W., Kindler, H., Stadler, W. M., Knowles, H. L., Bedrosian, C. & Ratain, M. J. (2009). A phase I trial to determine the safety, tolerability, and maximum tolerated dose of deforolimus in patients with advanced malignancies. *Clin Cancer Res,* Vol. 15, No. 4, pp. 1428-1434, ISSN 1078-0432 (Print)

Harzstark, A. L., Small, E. J., Weinberg, V. K., Sun, J., Ryan, C. J., Lin, A. M., Fong, L., Brocks, D. R. & Rosenberg, J. E. (2011). A phase 1 study of everolimus and sorafenib for metastatic clear cell renal cell carcinoma. *Cancer,* ISSN 0008-543X (Print)

Hay, N. & Sonenberg, N. (2004). Upstream and downstream of mTOR. *Genes Dev,* Vol. 18, No. 16, pp. 1926-1945, ISSN 0890-9369 (Print)

He, Y., Rajantie, I., Pajusola, K., Jeltsch, M., Holopainen, T., Yla-Herttuala, S., Harding, T., Jooss, K., Takahashi, T. & Alitalo, K. (2005). Vascular endothelial cell growth factor receptor 3-mediated activation of lymphatic endothelium is crucial for tumor cell entry and spread via lymphatic vessels. *Cancer Res,* Vol. 65, No. 11, pp. 4739-4746, ISSN 0008-5472 (Print)

Hirata, H., Hinoda, Y., Nakajima, K., Kawamoto, K., Kikuno, N., Kawakami, K., Yamamura, S., Ueno, K., Majid, S., Saini, S., Ishii, N. & Dahiya, R. (2009). Wnt antagonist gene DKK2 is epigenetically silenced and inhibits renal cancer progression through apoptotic and cell cycle pathways. *Clin Cancer Res,* Vol. 15, No. 18, pp. 5678-5687, ISSN 1078-0432 (Print)

Horie, S., Aruga, S., Kawamata, H., Okui, N., Kakizoe, T. & Kitamura, T. (1999). Biological role of HGF/MET pathway in renal cell carcinoma. *J Urol,* Vol. 161, No. 3, pp. 990-997, ISSN 0022-5347 (Print)

Hu-Lowe, D. D., Zou, H. Y., Grazzini, M. L., Hallin, M. E., Wickman, G. R., Amundson, K., Chen, J. H., Rewolinski, D. A., Yamazaki, S., Wu, E. Y., McTigue, M. A., Murray, B. W., Kania, R. S., O'Connor, P., Shalinsky, D. R. & Bender, S. L. (2008). Nonclinical antiangiogenesis and antitumor activities of axitinib (AG-013736), an oral, potent, and selective inhibitor of vascular endothelial growth factor receptor tyrosine kinases 1, 2, 3. *Clin Cancer Res,* Vol. 14, No. 22, pp. 7272-7283, ISSN 1078-0432 (Print)

Huang, H., Bhat, A., Woodnutt, G. & Lappe, R. (2010). Targeting the ANGPT-TIE2 pathway in malignancy. *Nat Rev Cancer,* Vol. 10, No. 8, pp. 575-585, ISSN 1474-1768 (Electronic)

Hudes, G., Carducci, M., Tomczak, P., Dutcher, J., Figlin, R., Kapoor, A., Staroslawska, E., Sosman, J., McDermott, D., Bodrogi, I., Kovacevic, Z., Lesovoy, V., Schmidt-Wolf, I. G., Barbarash, O., Gokmen, E., O'Toole, T., Lustgarten, S., Moore, L. & Motzer, R. J. (2007). Temsirolimus, interferon alfa, or both for advanced renal-cell carcinoma. *N Engl J Med,* Vol. 356, No. 22, pp. 2271-2281, ISSN 1533-4406 (Electronic)

Hudes, G. R., Berkenblit, A., Feingold, J., Atkins, M. B., Rini, B. I. & Dutcher, J. (2009). Clinical trial experience with temsirolimus in patients with advanced renal cell carcinoma. *Semin Oncol,* Vol. 36 Suppl 3, No. pp. S26-36, ISSN 1532-8708 (Electronic)

Inai, T., Mancuso, M., Hashizume, H., Baffert, F., Haskell, A., Baluk, P., Hu-Lowe, D. D., Shalinsky, D. R., Thurston, G., Yancopoulos, G. D. & McDonald, D. M. (2004). Inhibition of vascular endothelial growth factor (VEGF) signaling in cancer causes loss of endothelial fenestrations, regression of tumor vessels, and appearance of basement membrane ghosts. *Am J Pathol,* Vol. 165, No. 1, pp. 35-52, ISSN 0002-9440 (Print)

Inoki, K., Corradetti, M. N. & Guan, K. L. (2005). Dysregulation of the TSC-mTOR pathway in human disease. *Nat Genet,* Vol. 37, No. 1, pp. 19-24, ISSN 1061-4036 (Print)

Inoki, K., Ouyang, H., Zhu, T., Lindvall, C., Wang, Y., Zhang, X., Yang, Q., Bennett, C., Harada, Y., Stankunas, K., Wang, C. Y., He, X., MacDougald, O. A., You, M., Williams, B. O. & Guan, K. L. (2006). TSC2 integrates Wnt and energy signals via a coordinated phosphorylation by AMPK and GSK3 to regulate cell growth. *Cell,* Vol. 126, No. 5, pp. 955-968, ISSN 0092-8674 (Print)

Jain, R. K. (2005). Normalization of tumor vasculature: an emerging concept in antiangiogenic therapy. *Science,* Vol. 307, No. 5706, pp. 58-62, ISSN 1095-9203 (Electronic)

Jemal, A., Siegel, R., Ward, E., Hao, Y., Xu, J., Murray, T. & Thun, M. J. (2008). Cancer statistics, 2008. *CA Cancer J Clin,* Vol. 58, No. 2, pp. 71-96, ISSN 0007-9235 (Print)

Kataoka, Y., Mukohara, T., Tomioka, H., Funakoshi, Y., Kiyota, N., Fujiwara, Y., Yashiro, M., Hirakawa, K., Hirai, M. & Minami, H. (2011). Foretinib (GSK1363089), a multi-kinase inhibitor of MET and VEGFRs, inhibits growth of gastric cancer cell lines by blocking inter-receptor tyrosine kinase networks. *Invest New Drugs,* ISSN 1573-0646 (Electronic)

Kawakami, K., Hirata, H., Yamamura, S., Kikuno, N., Saini, S., Majid, S., Tanaka, Y., Kawamoto, K., Enokida, H., Nakagawa, M. & Dahiya, R. (2009). Functional significance of Wnt inhibitory factor-1 gene in kidney cancer. *Cancer Res,* Vol. 69, No. 22, pp. 8603-8610, ISSN 1538-7445 (Electronic)

Kim, E. S., Serur, A., Huang, J., Manley, C. A., McCrudden, K. W., Frischer, J. S., Soffer, S. Z., Ring, L., New, T., Zabski, S., Rudge, J. S., Holash, J., Yancopoulos, G. D., Kandel, J. J. & Yamashiro, D. J. (2002). Potent VEGF blockade causes regression of coopted vessels in a model of neuroblastoma. *Proc Natl Acad Sci U S A,* Vol. 99, No. 17, pp. 11399-11404, ISSN 0027-8424 (Print)

Klein, S. & Levitzki, A. (2009). Targeting the EGFR and the PKB pathway in cancer. *Curr Opin Cell Biol,* Vol. 21, No. 2, pp. 185-193, ISSN 1879-0410 (Electronic)

Koh, M. Y., Spivak-Kroizman, T., Venturini, S., Welsh, S., Williams, R. R., Kirkpatrick, D. L. & Powis, G. (2008). Molecular mechanisms for the activity of PX-478, an antitumor inhibitor of the hypoxia-inducible factor-1alpha. *Mol Cancer Ther,* Vol. 7, No. 1, pp. 90-100, ISSN 1535-7163 (Print)

Kojima, T., Shimazui, T., Hinotsu, S., Joraku, A., Oikawa, T., Kawai, K., Horie, R., Suzuki, H., Nagashima, R., Yoshikawa, K., Michiue, T., Asashima, M., Akaza, H. & Uchida, K. (2009). Decreased expression of CXXC4 promotes a malignant phenotype in renal cell carcinoma by activating Wnt signaling. *Oncogene,* Vol. 28, No. 2, pp. 297-305, ISSN 1476-5594 (Electronic)

Koochekpour, S., Jeffers, M., Wang, P. H., Gong, C., Taylor, G. A., Roessler, L. M., Stearman, R., Vasselli, J. R., Stetler-Stevenson, W. G., Kaelin, W. G., Jr., Linehan, W. M., Klausner, R. D., Gnarra, J. R. & Vande Woude, G. F. (1999). The von Hippel-Lindau tumor suppressor gene inhibits hepatocyte growth factor/scatter factor-induced invasion and branching morphogenesis in renal carcinoma cells. *Mol Cell Biol,* Vol. 19, No. 9, pp. 5902-5912, ISSN 0270-7306 (Print)

Kumar, R., Knick, V. B., Rudolph, S. K., Johnson, J. H., Crosby, R. M., Crouthamel, M. C., Hopper, T. M., Miller, C. G., Harrington, L. E., Onori, J. A., Mullin, R. J., Gilmer, T. M., Truesdale, A. T., Epperly, A. H., Boloor, A., Stafford, J. A., Luttrell, D. K. & Cheung, M. (2007). Pharmacokinetic-pharmacodynamic correlation from mouse to human with pazopanib, a multikinase angiogenesis inhibitor with potent antitumor and antiangiogenic activity. *Mol Cancer Ther,* Vol. 6, No. 7, pp. 2012-2021, ISSN 1535-7163 (Print)

Kummar, S., Gutierrez, M. E., Gardner, E. R., Chen, X., Figg, W. D., Zajac-Kaye, M., Chen, M., Steinberg, S. M., Muir, C. A., Yancey, M. A., Horneffer, Y. R., Juwara, L., Melillo, G., Ivy, S. P., Merino, M., Neckers, L., Steeg, P. S., Conley, B. A., Giaccone, G., Doroshow, J. H. & Murgo, A. J. (2010). Phase I trial of 17-dimethylaminoethylamino-17-demethoxygeldanamycin (17-DMAG), a heat shock protein inhibitor, administered twice weekly in patients with advanced malignancies. *Eur J Cancer,* Vol. 46, No. 2, pp. 340-347, ISSN 1879-0852 (Electronic)

Lang, J. M. & Harrison, M. R. (2010). Pazopanib for the treatment of patients with advanced renal cell carcinoma. *Clin Med Insights Oncol,* Vol. 4, No. pp. 95-105, ISSN 1179-5549 (Electronic)

Le Tourneau, C., Faivre, S., Serova, M. & Raymond, E. (2008). mTORC1 inhibitors: is temsirolimus in renal cancer telling us how they really work? *Br J Cancer,* Vol. 99, No. 8, pp. 1197-1203, ISSN 1532-1827 (Electronic)

Linehan, W. M., Rubin, J. S. & Bottaro, D. P. (2009). VHL loss of function and its impact on oncogenic signaling networks in clear cell renal cell carcinoma. *Int J Biochem Cell Biol,* Vol. 41, No. 4, pp. 753-756, ISSN 1878-5875 (Electronic)

Liu, J., Lin, T. H., Cole, A. G., Wen, R., Zhao, L., Brescia, M. R., Jacob, B., Hussain, Z., Appell, K. C., Henderson, I. & Webb, M. L. (2008). Identification and characterization of small-molecule inhibitors of Tie2 kinase. *FEBS Lett,* Vol. 582, No. 5, pp. 785-791, ISSN 0014-5793 (Print)

Mackenzie, M. J., Rini, B. I., Elson, P., Schwandt, A., Wood, L., Trinkhaus, M., Bjarnason, G. & Knox, J. (2011). Temsirolimus in VEGF-refractory metastatic renal cell carcinoma. *Ann Oncol,* Vol. 22, No. 1, pp. 145-148, ISSN 1569-8041 (Electronic)

Maira, S. M., Stauffer, F., Brueggen, J., Furet, P., Schnell, C., Fritsch, C., Brachmann, S., Chene, P., De Pover, A., Schoemaker, K., Fabbro, D., Gabriel, D., Simonen, M., Murphy, L., Finan, P., Sellers, W. & Garcia-Echeverria, C. (2008). Identification and characterization of NVP-BEZ235, a new orally available dual phosphatidylinositol 3-kinase/mammalian target of rapamycin inhibitor with potent in vivo antitumor activity. *Mol Cancer Ther,* Vol. 7, No. 7, pp. 1851-1863, ISSN 1535-7163 (Print)

Mamane, Y., Petroulakis, E., LeBacquer, O. & Sonenberg, N. (2006). mTOR, translation initiation and cancer. *Oncogene,* Vol. 25, No. 48, pp. 6416-6422, ISSN 0950-9232 (Print)

Mandriota, S. J., Turner, K. J., Davies, D. R., Murray, P. G., Morgan, N. V., Sowter, H. M., Wykoff, C. C., Maher, E. R., Harris, A. L., Ratcliffe, P. J. & Maxwell, P. H. (2002). HIF activation identifies early lesions in VHL kidneys: evidence for site-specific tumor suppressor function in the nephron. *Cancer Cell,* Vol. 1, No. 5, pp. 459-468, ISSN 1535-6108 (Print)

Maranchie, J. K., Vasselli, J. R., Riss, J., Bonifacino, J. S., Linehan, W. M. & Klausner, R. D. (2002). The contribution of VHL substrate binding and HIF1-alpha to the phenotype of VHL loss in renal cell carcinoma. *Cancer Cell,* Vol. 1, No. 3, pp. 247-255, ISSN 1535-6108 (Print)

Merseburger, A. S., Hennenlotter, J., Kuehs, U., Simon, P., Kruck, S., Koch, E., Stenzl, A. & Kuczyk, M. A. (2008). Activation of PI3K is associated with reduced survival in renal cell carcinoma. *Urol Int,* Vol. 80, No. 4, pp. 372-377, ISSN 1423-0399 (Electronic)

Miele, L., Golde, T. & Osborne, B. (2006). Notch signaling in cancer. *Curr Mol Med,* Vol. 6, No. 8, pp. 905-918, ISSN 1566-5240 (Print)

Miele, L., Miao, H. & Nickoloff, B. J. (2006). NOTCH signaling as a novel cancer therapeutic target. *Curr Cancer Drug Targets,* Vol. 6, No. 4, pp. 313-323, ISSN 1568-0096 (Print)

Moon, R. T., Kohn, A. D., De Ferrari, G. V. & Kaykas, A. (2004). WNT and beta-catenin signalling: diseases and therapies. *Nat Rev Genet,* Vol. 5, No. 9, pp. 691-701, ISSN 1471-0056 (Print)

Motzer, R. J., Hudes, G. R., Curti, B. D., McDermott, D. F., Escudier, B. J., Negrier, S., Duclos, B., Moore, L., O'Toole, T., Boni, J. P. & Dutcher, J. P. (2007b). Phase I/II trial of temsirolimus combined with interferon alfa for advanced renal cell carcinoma. *J Clin Oncol,* Vol. 25, No. 25, pp. 3958-3964, ISSN 1527-7755 (Electronic)

Motzer, R. J., Hutson, T. E., Tomczak, P., Michaelson, M. D., Bukowski, R. M., Oudard, S., Negrier, S., Szczylik, C., Pili, R., Bjarnason, G. A., Garcia-del-Muro, X., Sosman, J. A., Solska, E., Wilding, G., Thompson, J. A., Kim, S. T., Chen, I., Huang, X. & Figlin, R. A. (2009). Overall survival and updated results for sunitinib compared with interferon alfa in patients with metastatic renal cell carcinoma. *J Clin Oncol,* Vol. 27, No. 22, pp. 3584-3590, ISSN 1527-7755 (Electronic)

Motzer, R. J., Hutson, T. E., Tomczak, P., Michaelson, M. D., Bukowski, R. M., Rixe, O., Oudard, S., Negrier, S., Szczylik, C., Kim, S. T., Chen, I., Bycott, P. W., Baum, C. M. & Figlin, R. A. (2007a). Sunitinib versus interferon alfa in metastatic renal-cell carcinoma. *N Engl J Med,* Vol. 356, No. 2, pp. 115-124, ISSN 1533-4406 (Electronic)

Mulders, P. (2009). Vascular endothelial growth factor and mTOR pathways in renal cell carcinoma: differences and synergies of two targeted mechanisms. *BJU Int,* Vol. 104, No. 11, pp. 1585-1589, ISSN 1464-410X (Electronic)

Najafov, A., Sommer, E. M., Axten, J. M., Deyoung, M. P. & Alessi, D. R. (2010). Characterization of GSK2334470, a novel and highly specific inhibitor of PDK1. *Biochem J,* Vol. 433, No. 2, pp. 357-369, ISSN 1470-8728 (Electronic)

Nakamura, K., Taguchi, E., Miura, T., Yamamoto, A., Takahashi, K., Bichat, F., Guilbaud, N., Hasegawa, K., Kubo, K., Fujiwara, Y., Suzuki, R., Shibuya, M. & Isae, T. (2006). KRN951, a highly potent inhibitor of vascular endothelial growth factor receptor tyrosine kinases, has antitumor activities and affects functional vascular properties. *Cancer Res,* Vol. 66, No. 18, pp. 9134-9142, ISSN 0008-5472 (Print)

Natali, P. G., Prat, M., Nicotra, M. R., Bigotti, A., Olivero, M., Comoglio, P. M. & Di Renzo, M. F. (1996). Overexpression of the met/HGF receptor in renal cell carcinomas. *Int J Cancer,* Vol. 69, No. 3, pp. 212-217, ISSN 0020-7136 (Print)

Negrier, S., Gravis, G., Perol, D., Chevreau, C., Delva, R., Bay, J. O., Blanc, E., Ferlay, C., Geoffrois, L., Rolland, F., Legouffe, E., Sevin, E., Laguerre, B. & Escudier, B. (2011). Temsirolimus and bevacizumab, or sunitinib, or interferon alfa and bevacizumab for patients with advanced renal cell carcinoma (TORAVA): a randomised phase 2 trial. *Lancet Oncol,* ISSN 1474-5488 (Electronic)

Nickerson, M. L., Jaeger, E., Shi, Y., Durocher, J. A., Mahurkar, S., Zaridze, D., Matveev, V., Janout, V., Kollarova, H., Bencko, V., Navratilova, M., Szeszenia-Dabrowska, N., Mates, D., Mukeria, A., Holcatova, I., Schmidt, L. S., Toro, J. R., Karami, S., Hung, R., Gerard, G. F., Linehan, W. M., Merino, M., Zbar, B., Boffetta, P., Brennan, P., Rothman, N., Chow, W. H., Waldman, F. M. & Moore, L. E. (2008). Improved identification of von Hippel-Lindau gene alterations in clear cell renal tumors. *Clin Cancer Res,* Vol. 14, No. 15, pp. 4726-4734, ISSN 1078-0432 (Print)

Nickoloff, B. J., Osborne, B. A. & Miele, L. (2003). Notch signaling as a therapeutic target in cancer: a new approach to the development of cell fate modifying agents. *Oncogene,* Vol. 22, No. 42, pp. 6598-6608, ISSN 0950-9232 (Print)

Nicolas, M., Wolfer, A., Raj, K., Kummer, J. A., Mill, P., van Noort, M., Hui, C. C., Clevers, H., Dotto, G. P. & Radtke, F. (2003). Notch1 functions as a tumor suppressor in mouse skin. *Nat Genet,* Vol. 33, No. 3, pp. 416-421, ISSN 1061-4036 (Print)

O'Reilly, K. E., Rojo, F., She, Q. B., Solit, D., Mills, G. B., Smith, D., Lane, H., Hofmann, F., Hicklin, D. J., Ludwig, D. L., Baselga, J. & Rosen, N. (2006). mTOR inhibition induces upstream receptor tyrosine kinase signaling and activates Akt. *Cancer Res,* Vol. 66, No. 3, pp. 1500-1508, ISSN 0008-5472 (Print)

Oshiro, N., Yoshino, K., Hidayat, S., Tokunaga, C., Hara, K., Eguchi, S., Avruch, J. & Yonezawa, K. (2004). Dissociation of raptor from mTOR is a mechanism of rapamycin-induced inhibition of mTOR function. *Genes Cells,* Vol. 9, No. 4, pp. 359-366, ISSN 1356-9597 (Print)

Oudard, S., George, D., Medioni, J. & Motzer, R. (2007). Treatment options in renal cell carcinoma: past, present and future. *Ann Oncol,* Vol. 18 Suppl 10, pp. x25-31, ISSN 0923-7534 (Print)

Pal, S. K. & Figlin, R. A. (2011). Future directions of mammalian target of rapamycin (mTOR) inhibitor therapy in renal cell carcinoma. *Target Oncol,* Vol. 6, No. 1, pp. 5-16, ISSN 1776-260X (Electronic)

Pal, S. K., Kortylewski, M., Yu, H. & Figlin, R.A. (2010). Breaking through a plateau in renal cell carcinoma therapeutics: development and incorporation of biomarkers. Mol Cancer Ther, Vol. 9, No. 12, pp. 3115-25, ISSN 1538-8514 (Electronic)

Pantuck, A. J., Seligson, D. B., Klatte, T., Yu, H., Leppert, J. T., Moore, L., O'Toole, T., Gibbons, J., Belldegrun, A. S. & Figlin, R. A. (2007). Prognostic relevance of the mTOR pathway in renal cell carcinoma: implications for molecular patient selection for targeted therapy. *Cancer,* Vol. 109, No. 11, pp. 2257-2267, ISSN 0008-543X (Print)

Patel, N. S., Li, J. L., Generali, D., Poulsom, R., Cranston, D. W. & Harris, A. L. (2005). Up-regulation of delta-like 4 ligand in human tumor vasculature and the role of basal expression in endothelial cell function. *Cancer Res,* Vol. 65, No. 19, pp. 8690-8697, ISSN 0008-5472 (Print)

Patel, P. H., Senico, P. L., Curiel, R. E. & Motzer, R. J. (2009). Phase I study combining treatment with temsirolimus and sunitinib malate in patients with advanced renal cell carcinoma. *Clin Genitourin Cancer,* Vol. 7, No. 1, pp. 24-27, ISSN 1558-7673 (Print)

Peruzzi, B., Athauda, G. & Bottaro, D. P. (2006). The von Hippel-Lindau tumor suppressor gene product represses oncogenic beta-catenin signaling in renal carcinoma cells. *Proc Natl Acad Sci U S A,* Vol. 103, No. 39, pp. 14531-14536, ISSN 0027-8424 (Print)

Pietras, K., Sjoblom, T., Rubin, K., Heldin, C. H. & Ostman, A. (2003). PDGF receptors as cancer drug targets. *Cancer Cell,* Vol. 3, No. 5, pp. 439-443, ISSN 1535-6108 (Print)

Presta, L. G., Chen, H., O'Connor, S. J., Chisholm, V., Meng, Y. G., Krummen, L., Winkler, M. & Ferrara, N. (1997). Humanization of an anti-vascular endothelial growth factor monoclonal antibody for the therapy of solid tumors and other disorders. *Cancer Res,* Vol. 57, No. 20, pp. 4593-4599, ISSN 0008-5472 (Print)

Qian, C. N., Huang, D., Wondergem, B. & Teh, B. T. (2009). Complexity of tumor vasculature in clear cell renal cell carcinoma. *Cancer,* Vol. 115, No. 10 Suppl, pp. 2282-2289, ISSN 0008-543X (Print)

Rae, F. K., Stephenson, S. A., Nicol, D. L. & Clements, J. A. (2000). Novel association of a diverse range of genes with renal cell carcinoma as identified by differential display. *Int J Cancer,* Vol. 88, No. 5, pp. 726-732, ISSN 0020-7136 (Print)

Raval, R. R., Lau, K. W., Tran, M. G., Sowter, H. M., Mandriota, S. J., Li, J. L., Pugh, C. W., Maxwell, P. H., Harris, A. L. & Ratcliffe, P. J. (2005). Contrasting properties of hypoxia-inducible factor 1 (HIF-1) and HIF-2 in von Hippel-Lindau-associated renal cell carcinoma. *Mol Cell Biol,* Vol. 25, No. 13, pp. 5675-5686, ISSN 0270-7306 (Print)

Rixe, O., Bukowski, R. M., Michaelson, M. D., Wilding, G., Hudes, G. R., Bolte, O., Motzer, R. J., Bycott, P., Liau, K. F., Freddo, J., Trask, P. C., Kim, S. & Rini, B. I. (2007).

Axitinib treatment in patients with cytokine-refractory metastatic renal-cell cancer: a phase II study. *Lancet Oncol,* Vol. 8, No. 11, pp. 975-984, ISSN 1474-5488 (Electronic)

Ronnen, E. A., Kondagunta, G. V., Ishill, N., Sweeney, S. M., Deluca, J. K., Schwartz, L., Bacik, J. & Motzer, R. J. (2006). A phase II trial of 17-(Allylamino)-17-demethoxygeldanamycin in patients with papillary and clear cell renal cell carcinoma. *Invest New Drugs,* Vol. 24, No. 6, pp. 543-546, ISSN 0167-6997 (Print)

Ryan, C. W., Vuky, J., Chan, J. S., Chen, Z., Beer, T. M. & Nauman, D. (2011). A phase II study of everolimus in combination with imatinib for previously treated advanced renal carcinoma. *Invest New Drugs,* Vol. 29, No. 2, pp. 374-379, ISSN 1573-0646 (Electronic)

Sabatini, D. M. (2006). mTOR and cancer: insights into a complex relationship. *Nat Rev Cancer,* Vol. 6, No. 9, pp. 729-734, ISSN 1474-175X (Print)

Sansom, O. J., Griffiths, D. F., Reed, K. R., Winton, D. J. & Clarke, A. R. (2005). Apc deficiency predisposes to renal carcinoma in the mouse. *Oncogene,* Vol. 24, No. 55, pp. 8205-8210, ISSN 0950-9232 (Print)

Sarbassov, D. D., Ali, S. M., Sengupta, S., Sheen, J. H., Hsu, P. P., Bagley, A. F., Markhard, A. L. & Sabatini, D. M. (2006). Prolonged rapamycin treatment inhibits mTORC2 assembly and Akt/PKB. *Mol Cell,* Vol. 22, No. 2, pp. 159-168, ISSN 1097-2765 (Print)

Schmelzle, T. & Hall, M. N. (2000). TOR, a central controller of cell growth. *Cell,* Vol. 103, No. 2, pp. 253-262, ISSN 0092-8674 (Print)

Schoffski, P., Garcia, J. A., Stadler, W. M., Gil, T., Jonasch, E., Tagawa, S. T., Smitt, M., Yang, X., Oliner, K. S., Anderson, A., Zhu, M. & Kabbinavar, F. (2010). A phase II study of the efficacy and safety of AMG 102 in patients with metastatic renal cell carcinoma. *BJU Int,* ISSN 1464-410X (Electronic)

Shaw, R. J., Bardeesy, N., Manning, B. D., Lopez, L., Kosmatka, M., DePinho, R. A. & Cantley, L. C. (2004). The LKB1 tumor suppressor negatively regulates mTOR signaling. *Cancer Cell,* Vol. 6, No. 1, pp. 91-99, ISSN 1535-6108 (Print)

Sjolund, J., Johansson, M., Manna, S., Norin, C., Pietras, A., Beckman, S., Nilsson, E., Ljungberg, B. & Axelson, H. (2008). Suppression of renal cell carcinoma growth by inhibition of Notch signaling in vitro and in vivo. *J Clin Invest,* Vol. 118, No. 1, pp. 217-228, ISSN 0021-9738 (Print)

Slaton, J. W., Inoue, K., Perrotte, P., El-Naggar, A. K., Swanson, D. A., Fidler, I. J. & Dinney, C. P. (2001). Expression levels of genes that regulate metastasis and angiogenesis correlate with advanced pathological stage of renal cell carcinoma. *Am J Pathol,* Vol. 158, No. 2, pp. 735-743, ISSN 0002-9440 (Print)

Sosman, J. & Puzanov, I. (2009). Combination targeted therapy in advanced renal cell carcinoma. *Cancer,* Vol. 115, No. 10 Suppl, pp. 2368-2375, ISSN 0008-543X (Print)

Sosman, J. A., Flaherty, K.T., Atkins, M.B., et al. (2008). Updated results of phase I trial of sorafenib (S) and bevacizumab (B) in patients with metastatic renal cell cancer (mRCC) [abstract]. *J Clin Oncol,* Vol. 26(May 20 suppl)

Soulieres, D. (2009). Review of guidelines on the treatment of metastatic renal cell carcinoma. *Curr Oncol,* Vol. 16 Suppl 1, pp. S67-70, ISSN 1198-0052 (Print)

Sourbier, C., Lindner, V., Lang, H., Agouni, A., Schordan, E., Danilin, S., Rothhut, S., Jacqmin, D., Helwig, J. J. & Massfelder, T. (2006). The phosphoinositide 3-kinase/Akt pathway: a new target in human renal cell carcinoma therapy. *Cancer Res,* Vol. 66, No. 10, pp. 5130-5142, ISSN 0008-5472 (Print)

Staehler, M., Rohrmann, K., Haseke, N., Stief, C. G. & Siebels, M. (2005). Targeted agents for the treatment of advanced renal cell carcinoma. *Curr Drug Targets,* Vol. 6, No. 7, pp. 835-846, ISSN 1389-4501 (Print)

Sternberg, C. (2010). Randomized, Double-Blind Phase III Study Of Pazopanib In Patients With Advanced/Metastatic Renal Cell Carcinoma (mRCC): Final Overall Survival (OS) Results. *Ann Oncol,* Vol. 21, Abstract LBA22

Sternberg, C. N., Davis, I. D., Mardiak, J., Szczylik, C., Lee, E., Wagstaff, J., Barrios, C. H., Salman, P., Gladkov, O. A., Kavina, A., Zarba, J. J., Chen, M., McCann, L., Pandite, L., Roychowdhury, D. F. & Hawkins, R. E. (2010). Pazopanib in locally advanced or metastatic renal cell carcinoma: results of a randomized phase III trial. *J Clin Oncol,* Vol. 28, No. 6, pp. 1061-1068, ISSN 1527-7755 (Electronic)

Sulzbacher, I., Birner, P., Traxler, M., Marberger, M. & Haitel, A. (2003). Expression of platelet-derived growth factor-alpha alpha receptor is associated with tumor progression in clear cell renal cell carcinoma. *Am J Clin Pathol,* Vol. 120, No. 1, pp. 107-112, ISSN 0002-9173 (Print)

Takeda, M., Arao, T., Yokote, H., Komatsu, T., Yanagihara, K., Sasaki, H., Yamada, Y., Tamura, T., Fukuoka, K., Kimura, H., Saijo, N. & Nishio, K. (2007). AZD2171 shows potent antitumor activity against gastric cancer over-expressing fibroblast growth factor receptor 2/keratinocyte growth factor receptor. *Clin Cancer Res,* Vol. 13, No. 10, pp. 3051-3057, ISSN 1078-0432 (Print)

Tanimoto, S., Fukumori, T., El-Moula, G., Shiirevnyamba, A., Kinouchi, S., Koizumi, T., Nakanishi, R., Yamamoto, Y., Taue, R., Yamaguchi, K., Nakatsuji, H., Kishimoto, T., Izaki, H., Oka, N., Takahashi, M. & Kanayama, H. O. (2008). Prognostic significance of serum hepatocyte growth factor in clear cell renal cell carcinoma: comparison with serum vascular endothelial growth factor. *J Med Invest,* Vol. 55, No. 1-2, pp. 106-111, ISSN 1343-1420 (Print)

Thomas, G. V., Tran, C., Mellinghoff, I. K., Welsbie, D. S., Chan, E., Fueger, B., Czernin, J. & Sawyers, C. L. (2006). Hypoxia-inducible factor determines sensitivity to inhibitors of mTOR in kidney cancer. *Nat Med,* Vol. 12, No. 1, pp. 122-127, ISSN 1078-8956 (Print)

Thoreen, C. C., Kang, S. A., Chang, J. W., Liu, Q., Zhang, J., Gao, Y., Reichling, L. J., Sim, T., Sabatini, D. M. & Gray, N. S. (2009). An ATP-competitive mammalian target of rapamycin inhibitor reveals rapamycin-resistant functions of mTORC1. *J Biol Chem,* Vol. 284, No. 12, pp. 8023-8032, ISSN 0021-9258 (Print)

Toschi, L. & Janne, P. A. (2008). Single-agent and combination therapeutic strategies to inhibit hepatocyte growth factor/MET signaling in cancer. *Clin Cancer Res,* Vol. 14, No. 19, pp. 5941-5946, ISSN 1078-0432 (Print)

Uemura, H., Fujimoto, K., Tanaka, M., Yoshikawa, M., Hirao, Y., Uejima, S., Yoshikawa, K. & Itoh, K. (2006). A phase I trial of vaccination of CA9-derived peptides for HLA-

A24-positive patients with cytokine-refractory metastatic renal cell carcinoma. *Clin Cancer Res,* Vol. 12, No. 6, pp. 1768-1775, ISSN 1078-0432 (Print)

Veronese, M. L., Mosenkis, A., Flaherty, K. T., Gallagher, M., Stevenson, J. P., Townsend, R. R. & O'Dwyer, P. J. (2006). Mechanisms of hypertension associated with BAY 43-9006. *J Clin Oncol,* Vol. 24, No. 9, pp. 1363-1369, ISSN 1527-7755 (Electronic)

Vickers, M. M. & Heng, D.Y. (2010). Prognostic and predictive biomarkers in renal cell carcinoma. *Target Oncol,* Vol. 5, No. 2, pp. 85-94, ISSN 1776-260X (Electronic)

Wilhelm, S. M., Adnane, L., Newell, P., Villanueva, A., Llovet, J. M. & Lynch, M. (2008). Preclinical overview of sorafenib, a multikinase inhibitor that targets both Raf and VEGF and PDGF receptor tyrosine kinase signaling. *Mol Cancer Ther,* Vol. 7, No. 10, pp. 3129-3140, ISSN 1535-7163 (Print)

Wilhelm, S. M., Carter, C., Tang, L., Wilkie, D., McNabola, A., Rong, H., Chen, C., Zhang, X., Vincent, P., McHugh, M., Cao, Y., Shujath, J., Gawlak, S., Eveleigh, D., Rowley, B., Liu, L., Adnane, L., Lynch, M., Auclair, D., Taylor, I., Gedrich, R., Voznesensky, A., Riedl, B., Post, L. E., Bollag, G. & Trail, P. A. (2004). BAY 43-9006 exhibits broad spectrum oral antitumor activity and targets the RAF/MEK/ERK pathway and receptor tyrosine kinases involved in tumor progression and angiogenesis. *Cancer Res,* Vol. 64, No. 19, pp. 7099-7109, ISSN 0008-5472 (Print)

Wright, T. M., Brannon, A. R., Gordan, J. D., Mikels, A. J., Mitchell, C., Chen, S., Espinosa, I., van de Rijn, M., Pruthi, R., Wallen, E., Edwards, L., Nusse, R. & Rathmell, W. K. (2009). Ror2, a developmentally regulated kinase, promotes tumor growth potential in renal cell carcinoma. *Oncogene,* Vol. 28, No. 27, pp. 2513-2523, ISSN 1476-5594 (Electronic)

Wulff, C., Wilson, H., Wiegand, S. J., Rudge, J. S. & Fraser, H. M. (2002). Prevention of thecal angiogenesis, antral follicular growth, and ovulation in the primate by treatment with vascular endothelial growth factor Trap R1R2. *Endocrinology,* Vol. 143, No. 7, pp. 2797-2807, ISSN 0013-7227 (Print)

Xia, X., Qian, S., Soriano, S., Wu, Y., Fletcher, A. M., Wang, X. J., Koo, E. H., Wu, X. & Zheng, H. (2001). Loss of presenilin 1 is associated with enhanced beta-catenin signaling and skin tumorigenesis. *Proc Natl Acad Sci U S A,* Vol. 98, No. 19, pp. 10863-10868, ISSN 0027-8424 (Print)

Yamazaki, S., Skaptason, J., Romero, D., Vekich, S., Jones, H. M., Tan, W., Wilner, K. D. & Koudriakova, T. (2011). Prediction of oral pharmacokinetics of cMet kinase inhibitors in humans: physiologically based pharmacokinetic model versus traditional one-compartment model. *Drug Metab Dispos,* Vol. 39, No. 3, pp. 383-393, ISSN 1521-009X (Electronic)

Yu, K., Shi, C., Toral-Barza, L., Lucas, J., Shor, B., Kim, J. E., Zhang, W. G., Mahoney, R., Gaydos, C., Tardio, L., Kim, S. K., Conant, R., Curran, K., Kaplan, J., Verheijen, J., Ayral-Kaloustian, S., Mansour, T. S., Abraham, R. T., Zask, A. & Gibbons, J. J. (2010). Beyond rapalog therapy: preclinical pharmacology and antitumor activity of WYE-125132, an ATP-competitive and specific inhibitor of mTORC1 and mTORC2. *Cancer Res,* Vol. 70, No. 2, pp. 621-631, ISSN 1538-7445 (Electronic)

Zbar, B., Klausner, R. & Linehan, W. M. (2003). Studying cancer families to identify kidney cancer genes. *Annu Rev Med,* Vol. 54, No. pp. 217-233, ISSN 0066-4219 (Print)

Zhou, Y. D., Kim, Y. P., Mohammed, K. A., Jones, D. K., Muhammad, I., Dunbar, D. C. & Nagle, D. G. (2005). Terpenoid tetrahydroisoquinoline alkaloids emetine, klugine, and isocephaeline inhibit the activation of hypoxia-inducible factor-1 in breast tumor cells. *J Nat Prod,* Vol. 68, No. 6, pp. 947-950, ISSN 0163-3864 (Print)